B&T.
2 8. 85
9/上刊15

The
DILEMMA
of the FETUS

FETAL RESEARCH

MEDICAL PROGRESS

AND MORAL POLITICS

The
DILEMMA
of the FETUS

FETAL RESEARCH

MEDICAL PROGRESS

AND MORAL POLITICS

Steven Maynard-Moody

ST. MARTIN'S PRESS
NEW YORK

Design by Sara Stemen

ISBN 0-312-11785-X

First Edition: April 1995

10   9   8   7   6   5   4   3   2   1

For Carey

Acknowledgments

In countless ways, both large and small, many people have helped me in my journey through this book. Guy and Terri Walden willingly discussed their personal experiences as parents of a child who received a fetus-to-fetus tissue transplant; I hope I have done justice to their poignant story. Most of the research for this book was done in the various libraries of the University of Kansas, whose reference librarians helped me find my way through the maze of government and scientific materials. Some of my most interesting days of research were spent in the Clendening History of Medicine Library at the University of Kansas Medical Center, where Susan Case, the rare books librarian, was a constant source of good leads, much help, and interesting conversation.

Carey Maynard-Moody, George Frederickson, Elaine Sharp, Thelma Helyer, and Elizabeth Stella read and commented on several chapters. Marisa Kelly, Dvora Yanow, and Allan Hanson reviewed my entire manuscript, suggesting numerous improvements. Robert Weil and Becky Koh, my editors at St. Martin's Press, greatly strengthened this book with their guidance, encouragement, and suggestions.

This book and I owe a special debt to Dorothy Nelkin, University Professor of Sociology and Law, New York University. In the late 1970s, I was Dot's research assistant while a graduate student at Cornell University. She first suggested that I examine the then nascent fetal research controversy, research that ended in my first publication. Dot's help went far beyond that of a teacher, however. In her many books, she has provided a model for scholars who want to write about difficult and important issues with the clarity and strength needed to engage a general audience. In more personal ways, she helped me through the difficult early stages of this book by encouraging me to refine my ideas and clarify the themes, and she read and commented liberally on the first eight chapters of the manuscript. Without Dot's guidance, inspiration, and generosity, I doubt I would have focused on this topic, would have been able to think clearly about these issues, or would have had the courage to write this book.

And so, thanks to all who have helped and supported me. I hope I can repay your many kindnesses.

Contents

Illustrations

Preface

I first started thinking about the ideas expressed in this book in the late 1970s while a graduate student at Cornell University. As a research assistant in the Science, Technology, and Society Program, I was assigned the task of reading through the recombinant DNA hearings of the Cambridge City Council, a tedious task only a doctoral student could love. Recombinant DNA, or gene-splicing, had just become controversial. Some scientists saw great promise in this new technique of cutting and pasting fragments of genetic code. Other scientists, environmental groups, and the lay public feared that genetic engineers would unwittingly create and release deadly man-made microbes against which animals and plants would have no natural resistance. Some critics of recombinant DNA raised philosophical qualms about swapping genetic material across species; they believed that scientists should keep their hands off the code of creation.

When the Harvard Biology Department decided, although

not unanimously, to renovate an old lab to meet the safety standards required to conduct gene-splicing research, the city of Cambridge, Massachusetts, declared a moratorium on the research and held public hearings on the value and safety of the recombinant DNA. Although Cambridge is home to Harvard and the Massachusetts Institute of Technology, its city government does not reflect these elite research universities. Its mayor and city council were not scientists or scholars but the same kind of activist citizens that make up local governments across the country. In Cambridge they represented more the blue-collar locals than the lab-coated scientists, yet these local politicians took on the same issues that blue-ribbon panels of scientists and the National Institutes of Health had confronted.

As I perused the two and a half inches of transcripts I sensed an important transformation. These hearings began with much distrust between scientists and politicians: the scientists felt that the city council had no right to tell them what research they could and could not do and the city council feared both the unspecified risk of microscopic Frankensteins escaping the labs and their own inability to deal with complex scientific questions. But as the hearings proceeded anger and fear gave way to co-operation and a growing sense of competence. The scientists discovered that these politicians were not "know-nothings" out to halt research, and the politicians discovered that while they may not understand the technical details of recombinant DNA, they could sensibly deal with the broad social issues involved in this new technology. As a student of government, I sensed, although in a diffuse way, that something important had occurred in those city council hearings; it was a glimpse of how democratic forums could respond to complex scientific issues.

My next graduate student project was to write a chapter on the then-young dispute surrounding fetal research for a book devoted to controversies about science (Dorothy Nelkin, editor, *Controversy: The Politics of Technical Decisions,* Beverly Hills, CA: Sage Publications, 1979), a dispute that raised many of the same issues as the recombinant DNA hearings but one that proved to have no lasting resolution. Through the 1980s, my attention turned to other policy and scholarly interests but the questions posed by fetal research continued to nag at my thoughts. Questions of science and technology rarely get much attention except when new advances are announced, yet I felt that the issues posed by fetal research and other areas of science were far more socially significant than most of the issues that crowd the political agenda. As I twice revised my chapter for the second and third editions of *Controversy,* I became convinced that the protracted, seemingly endless dispute over fetal research and now fetal tissue transplantation was a contemporary morality play telling of the complex relationship of science, society, and government. It touched on the ancient tension between progress and tradition, was impelled by the conflicting moral claims of scientists and antiabortionists, and showed our struggle to come to grips with science-induced changes in our sense of who we are as individuals.

Over the decade of the 1980s, the more I looked at this political dispute the more fascinated I became. I wanted to learn more about the moral politics of science and followed the path that most helps me learn—I wrote. As this book leaves my hands and enters yours, I only hope that regardless of your initial position or views, you can confront the essential complexity of the issues involved and can do so with the belief that our cherished, if much maligned, democratic institutions will serve us only if we allow them to address the important dilemmas of our day, including those implied in scientific advance.

In chronicling the collision of moral politics and fetal research, this book examines several issues:

- How advances in knowledge and medical practice are changing our idea of fetal "personhood"
- How antiabortion groups transformed an obscure area of medical research into a sustained political conflict
- How moral politics have changed research decisions

and strained the cooperative relationship between
science and government
  • How government institutions failed to find and en-
    force a resolution of this controversy

After introducing the main themes, the book looks back at
the first public dispute over fetal research in Chapter 1. This
chapter begins before this research became controversial and
describes the first protest by antiabortionists over the use of
live fetuses as research subjects. Chapters 2 and 3 examine the
various forms of fetal research. Fetal research encompasses a
wide array of studies, from routine autopsies to science-fiction-
like fetal tissue transplants. These different forms of research,
discoveries about the fetus, and changing medical practices are
forcing us to reconsider the meaning of fetal life and the status
of the fetus, the subjects of Chapter 4.

Ambiguity about the meaning of fetal life and the status of
the fetus has also generated conflicting images of the fetus,
images that foster irreconcilable differences. Those who view
the fetus as maternal tissue cannot find common ground with
those who see it as a baby. Chapters 5 and 6 examine these and
other images of the fetus and discuss how they define the fetus's
cultural and social status. Chapter 7 looks at the ethical issues
raised by fetal research and its reliance on abortion for scientific
control and as a source of tissue.

Chapter 8 returns to the events in the controversy. The first
phase of the controversy ended in the mid-1970s with the federal government rejecting all limits on fetal research, even those
proposed by the experts serving on the first national commission. This initial resolution did not hold, however. Chapters 9,
10, and 11 examine how the fetal research controversy evolved
as the White House, Congress, the science bureaucracies, and
additional national commissions took up the issues but repeatedly failed to find a solution that permitted progress but gave
voice to moral fears.

This policy stalemate was eventually broken, not by resolving
the issues at the heart of this conflict, but when the pull of

progress overwhelmed moral restraint. Chapters 12 and 13 discuss how as research progressed from the abstract realm of discovery to the tangible realm of treatment the fetal research opponents lost influence. The irresistible pull of progress, in the end, trumps moral concerns about the processes and implications of scientific discovery.

Public controversy with its overheated rhetoric, chaotic history, and seemingly pointless repetition is, to many, emblematic of the failure of our government to deal with difficult contemporary problems. The book ends with a different conclusion. The epilogue examines the positive role of science controversies in democratic control over science policy.

As this book goes to press in January 1995, fetal research is once again becoming controversial. In November 1994, Republicans won, for the first time in forty years, majorities in both the House and Senate. The antiabortion members of Congress counted many newly elected representatives as allies and announced that they would reverse the Clinton administration's permission for medical research that is related to abortion, such as fetal tissue transplantation and the abortion pill RU-486. Right-wing Representative Robert Dornan (Republican, California) declared that "We will systematically undo . . . those five in-your-face executive orders . . ." signed with much fanfare by President Clinton on his first day in office, which allowed federal funding of human fetal tissue transplantation research. "I expect we're going to be fighting all those fights [over fetal research] all over again," lamented profetal research Representative Henry Waxman (Democrat, California).

Then, after overturning Presidents Reagan's and Bush's bans on fetal tissue transplantation and denouncing his predecessors for politicizing science, President Clinton recently followed their lead: he rejected the advice of an embryo advisory panel and prohibited the National Institutes of Health from funding research that involved creating human embryos. Patricia King, a law professor and panel co-chair, denounced Clinton's decision as having more to do with "politics" than with the "merits of embryo research."

Thus, although the issues may change, the conflict between scientific progress and moral politics endures because the difficult and painful issues at the heart of fetal research remain unresolved. As we stand on a threshold looking back over twenty years of controversy over fetal research and looking forward to a future of mounting conflict over new areas of science—embryology, human cloning, genetic engineering, to name just a few—the issues examined in this book are ever more poignant.

The DILEMMA *of the* FETUS

FETAL RESEARCH

MEDICAL PROGRESS

AND MORAL POLITICS

Introduction

On January 22, 1993, within a day of taking office, President Clinton rescinded former President Bush's 1989 executive order that banned federal funding for fetal tissue transplantation research.[1] Despite promises of miracle cures and the pleading of experts in favor of fetal research, antiabortion activists in the Bush administration had starved fetal transplant research by cutting off its access to federal money.[2] Fetal tissue transplants depend on abortion, and anything associated with abortion was anathema to this group. The issue was rarely mentioned during the 1992 presidential campaign, but the ban on funding for fetal research symbolized to the Clinton administration the poisonous dominance of ideology over science.

President Clinton's executive order marked the end of the most recent stage in a twenty-year controversy over fetal research, but the issues that fueled this protracted conflict continue to smolder. To research supporters, the ban was a dangerous intrusion of politics into the almost sacred, if aseptic, preserve of science. To fetal research opponents, Clinton's order and the renewal of fetal research tell of the relentless crushing of morals and traditional values by the bulldozer of scientific "progress."

On the surface, the fetal research controversy is kindled by the connection of fetal research and abortion. The controversy began in 1973 after the *Roe* v. *Wade* ruling galvanized opposition to abortion. The fetal research dispute cannot, however, be reduced to a simple conflict of interests; it is more than a conflict between antiabortionists and scientists, between anti-research traditionalists and pro-research progressives. The issues raised by this dispute tell of the ambivalent place of science in our culture. Political conflicts over science are the bubbles in a boiling pot; they are the surface events, but the source of heat that brings these issues to boil is the friction between our addiction to progress and our fear that science erodes human values.

This is an ancient tension, and at its core the fetal research controversy is a contemporary version of the tragedy of Faust, the medieval scientist who sold his soul to the devil to gain forbidden knowledge. Dr. Faust dreams of the power, accomplishment, and eternal recognition of medical advancement; a dream that echoes today in labs throughout the world. Faust makes a pact with the devil and achieves his dream, but at a cost. To learn forbidden knowledge and gain forbidden power, he must give up what is uniquely human, his soul.

In the case of fetal research, no one doubts the value of the knowledge gained or the cures promised. Surely the prevention of birth defects, the deepening of understanding of fetal development, and the almost magical cures promised by fetal tissue transplants add immeasurably to the quality of our lives. But like the Faust legend, the fetal research controversy shows how, in the late twentieth century, we are drawn to knowledge and technical advance and yet are torn about their social and human costs. Popular media images of scientists show traces of the Faust legend and our discomfort with science's unbridled power. Scientists are often portrayed as driven by an "ungovernable instinct to extend the boundaries of knowledge"[3]; an instinct admired yet feared.

The fetal research controversy arose because of moral concerns about the process of discovery. The controversy concerns the research itself, not the uses of the research. On one level, these concerns reflect difficult practical and ethical questions about the involvement of human fetuses in biomedical research. Much fetal research stretches, if not breaks, the codes of research ethics that guide human experimentation, leaving some to conclude that such research should not proceed. Others observe that an undeveloped fetus is not a "human research subject"—it is tissue, not a person—and that therefore norms of research ethics do not apply.

On a deeper level, the discoveries of fetal research are forcing us to rethink difficult and unsettling value questions. New discoveries about fetal development and advances in fetal diagnosis and imaging challenge long-held assumptions about when the rapidly developing fetus becomes a person and what, if any, rights it can claim. New forms of fetal therapy and surgery are elevating the status of the fetus to that of a patient separate from the mother. This new status creates the potential for conflict between a woman's right to bodily autonomy and a fetus's right to treatment.

Although these and other issues are often obscured by the technical jargon of scientists and the moral hyperbole of abortion opponents, fetal research raises questions about who we are and what we value. The fetal research controversy is based on our struggle to find answers to such questions, and when different groups within our society reach irreconcilable conclusions, it tells of our struggle to deal with our differences.

Fetal research was not, of course, the only area of science caught in social and political controversy.[4] Over the past twenty years, protests have erupted over such uses of science as nuclear power, and over the risks associated with such advances as gene-splicing and genetically altered food. Ozone holes, endangered species, DNA testing, genetically engineered cow hormones— the list of public controversies over science grows almost weekly.

Amid this chorus of protest over the uses and risks of science, research and the process of discovery for the most part have remained sheltered in a state of political grace. Research is funded and supported by government, but researchers are allowed, even encouraged, to follow their own interests and priorities. Many believe that generous support and the unbridled freedom of inquiry are the essential ingredients to scientific and social progress.[5]

Prior to 1973, fetal researchers followed many lines of inquiry with the blessing of federal grants. In the 1960s, fetal research was an exciting field; it attracted ambitious, creative researchers who anticipated careers of important discoveries and major contributions to prenatal health. After fetal research became controversial, federal funding withered and scientific excitement soured.

The negative effects of social controversy on science is ironic because science itself progresses through controversy. Heated, often rancorous debates lead to new ways of thinking and discovery. These disputes among scientists are acceptable, even desirable, to fellow scientists; they are part of the culture of science. Controversies over science, especially over the process of research, that spill out of the scientific community are, on the other hand, shocking and abhorrent to most scientists.[5] This response to controversies over science reflects the strongly held and widely shared belief in the absolute freedom of inquiry.

Most scientists believe that while the products of science can be used for good or evil, the process of science is itself pure.[6] Research on the structure of matter, in this view, remains untarnished regardless of how grotesque the results of the atom bomb or how dangerous the storage of atomic waste. While government can and must regulate the products of research, in the views of many scientists it must keep its distance from research itself. As Hans Jonas comments, "Freedom in inquiry is claimed, granted, and cherished as unqualified on the premise that inquiry as such raises no moral problems."[7]

The belief that research, although not its applications, is neutral and must be protected constitutes a basic tenet of what Robert Proctor calls the political ideology of science.[8] In this view, science itself is "value-free" and "values or politics enter only as contamination."[9] As the power and stature of science has grown over the past 150 years, this political ideology has become a cornerstone of modern societies. It was not always so, and, as controversies such as the one over fetal research tell us, it may not always be so. But the belief that inquiry is sacrosanct is central to the cultural authority and political autonomy of science. Supporters of scientific autonomy argue that physical, material, and cultural progress are threatened if science is guided by anything but itself.

This argument extends to democracy itself. The political ideology of science asserts that free science is necessary for a free society; research freedom, like free speech and a free press, is, in this view, a fundamental right.[10] Even more than a fundamental right, scientific research—because of its relentless questioning of accepted wisdom—actively promotes freedom by continuously challenging tyrannies of all sorts, from entrenched theories to accepted ideologies. The caption under a portrait of Benjamin Franklin, the archetype of the scientist democrat, expresses this dual role: "He wrested the lightning from the sky and the scepter from the Tyrants."[11]

The fetal research controversy challenged the political ideology of science; it undermined science's legitimacy and authority. During the fetal research controversy, science, or at least this one form of science, fell from its state of grace. It was no longer protected from political intrusion; research became just one more government program subject to the same political concerns and ploys as other programs. Congress began to look at scientists "as just another selfish pressure group, not as the wizards of perpetual progress."[12]

Moral concerns about the process of research created the fetal research dispute, but doubts and restraints could not, in the end, stand against the tide of medical progress. As fetal research moved from promise toward treatment, from the lab to the doctor's office, controversy lost its grip. The good ends of medical advance may not justify questionable means, but, once achieved, good ends do allow us to forget the means. If the fetal research testing the German measles vaccine and amniocentesis aroused concern, once proven safe we are still glad to use them. We are collectively willing to halt unproven fetal tissue transplants, but as soon as they become an established cure for diabetes or Parkinson's disease such restraint will vanish.

Social controversies over science do express our doubts and discomforts, but they have only frayed the edges of the fabric of our belief in science and technology. Many scholars have written of the growth of antiscience sentiment, the general decline of professional authority, and the increase in "nonmaterialist and noninstrumental" orientations.[13] On the surface, the fetal research controversy supports this argument: research opponents expressed vehement antiscience views. On a deeper level, however, the fetal research controversy underscores our devotion to scientific progress, for in the end, despite unresolved and perhaps unresolvable doubts, the relentless pull of progress overwhelmed resistance to the research.

The fetal research controversy also has important implications for governing in the late twentieth century. Even though the federal funding bans were eventually lifted, scientists see this twenty-year controversy as a horror story. To them it is a nightmarish intrusion of politics into science and a violation of the basic freedom of inquiry. To opponents of fetal research, however, Clinton's lifting of the ban represents one more failure in their just battle to assert that moral claims and traditional values must take precedence over all else, including scientific progress. To others not caught in the fray, the fetal research conflict reflects the gridlock and cowardice of contemporary government; more evidence that "In contemporary America, officials do not govern, they merely posture."[14] This conflict, as we shall see, was socially divisive without leading to a resolution of the issues; it generated much political heat but little policy light.

Against this generalized disgust with the process and results of the fetal research controversy—everyone involved was dissatisfied—I propose what must seem like an audacious argument: Social and political conflict over science is essential and healthy. Most of us readily agree with Robert Proctor that "Science is the product of society and must remain accountable to that society."[15] Conflict, and the ever-present potential for conflict, is essential to sustaining the social accountability of science. Any process or procedure that reduces conflict over science weakens social control; without conflict scientists rule science policy, during conflict their dominance is, at least momentarily, diminished.

This dispute, with all its loose ends and disruption, did force scientists, protesters, and government officials to confront basic issues that had previously been overlooked. The often bitter and unproductive dispute over fetal research enlarged our capacity to face such controversies. At a minimum, science controversies broaden the groups represented and the issues discussed. Controversy creates a public stage on which different values and issues are expressed. It changes the language of science decision making from the technical and exclusionary terms of experts to the cruder, if more participatory, dialect of politics. Controversy also forces the press, which tends to fawn over discovery and scientists, to present a less one-sided pro-science view.[16]

To face controversial issues does not necessarily mean that we can resolve them, either by finding a solution acceptable to opposing interests or by the brute force of government authority. But, however frustrated the opposing groups and the public may be by our collective inability to resolve controversial issues, this failure is trivial compared to the failure of avoidance.

To avoid facing the issues raised by fetal research, as was the case before the conflict began, is far more dangerous than our inability to resolve them. Nearly thirty years ago, Jacob Bronowski wrote, "The world today is made, it is powered by science; and for any man to abdicate an interest in science is to walk with eyes open toward slavery."[17] Bronowski was overly optimistic. Without public engagement in the social and moral issues that are implicit in science, we are walking with eyes closed toward slavery. Controversy, as unwelcome as it so often is, opens our eyes.

1 From the Laboratory to the Streets

The Foreshocks of the Fetal Research

Controversy in the Years

Leading up to Roe *v.* Wade

etal research was important to medical science long before it became controversial, long before it was caught in the storm of moral politics. In 1928, Italian researchers transplanted human fetal pancreas tissue into a patient suffering from diabetes, and eleven years later researchers in the U.S. repeated the operation; none of the patients in these experiments improved. Fetal tissue did, however, play a role in one of the century's medical breakthroughs: the Salk antipolio vaccine, which ended the dreaded polio epidemic, was developed in the early 1950s in part using human fetal kidney cells.

It was a medical disaster, however, that spurred an active program of fetal research.[1] In 1957, a German drug company began marketing tranquilizers and sleeping pills containing thalidomide. This non-habit-forming pill was considered so safe that in some countries it was sold without prescription. By 1960, Germans, including pregnant women, were taking 15 million thalidomide pills per month. U.S. sales, however, were blocked by a skeptical Food and Drug Administration pharmacologist, Dr. Frances Kelsey. Drug companies were furious that a federal bureaucrat could block approval of this seemingly safe and effective drug, but Kelsey had a hunch that the safety research was not telling the whole story. The pill did not harm the research animals, but neither did it tranquilize them.[2]

Meanwhile, between 1959 and 1961, European doctors noted with growing alarm an epidemic among newborns of phocomelia, or "seal-limbs"—an unprecedented number of babies were born with stumps instead of arms and legs. In 1961, a German physician suggested a connection between phocomelia and thalidomide, a connection that was quickly confirmed. Most of the nearly 5,000 cases of phocomelia occurred in Europe, where thalidomide was legal. A few cases appeared in the U.S. when doctors handed out trial doses distributed by drug companies or from pills brought in from Europe.[3]

One Arizona mother of four, Sherri Finkbine, discovered that she was taking thalidomide while pregnant; her husband had brought the prescription back from London. Fearing giving birth to a deformed child, she decided to have an abortion. Mrs. Finkbine, a local TV moderator of the children's show *Romper Room,* also decided to discuss her situation publicly to forewarn other mothers. The county prosecutor then announced that he would charge Mrs. Finkbine if she had the abortion; prior to *Roe* v. *Wade* abortion was illegal in Arizona unless the pregnant woman's life was at risk. After several court hearings and mounting publicity, she had her abortion abroad.

For several years prior to the thalidomide disaster, Tennessee senator Estes Kefauver had been unsuccessfully advocating more stringent testing and controls over drugs. The public fear of dangerous drugs aroused by thalidomide—the fear that a drug considered harmless could cause such devastating and unexpected deformities to helpless newborns—created the political support needed to pass the Kefauver–Harris Amendments to the Federal Food, Drug, and Cosmetics Act.[4] These amendments required pharmaceutical companies to determine if drugs were safe and effective before they were distributed to the public. To prevent future thalidomide disasters, drug companies would need to show that new drugs and antibiotics were safe to the developing fetus before they could be prescribed to pregnant women. The thalidomide disaster clearly demonstrated that animal studies were not sufficient to prove safety to the fetus.

Spurred by the need to test the safety of medication on the fetus, fetal research became increasingly common and ever more important to medical science during the 1960s. This was also a time when, increasingly, planned abortions were taking place in hospitals, where fetal remains were readily available to researchers.[5] By the early 1970s, fetal research was a hot scientific area with importance extending well beyond the testing of new drugs. It already had produced important medical advances and promised many more. For the first time, doctors could reliably diagnose mother-fetus blood incompatibility, or Rh disease. Progress was made in the neonatal treatment of respiratory distress. Amniocentesis and prenatal genetic screening emerged from experimental testing to become routine practice. Young medical researchers entered the field looking forward to interesting and productive careers. Prior to 1973 and the *Roe* v. *Wade* decision, research that would later spark public controversy was quietly planned, funded, completed, and published without evoking a hint of public concern.

For example, in the early 1970s, scientists used living but nonviable fetuses to test new systems of fetal life support—creating, in effect, an artificial placenta that would enable doctors to keep very young fetuses alive. As discussed in detail later, "nonviable" is a medical term for a fetus that shows some life signs, such as heartbeat, but is too undeveloped to survive for long outside the womb. In one experiment, eight living but nonviable fetuses were obtained by hysterotomy, a procedure similar to a cesarean delivery. Right after the operation small tubes were inserted in the umbilical arteries and veins for pumping and removing oxygenated blood. These tiny fetuses—they

weighed between 300 and 980 grams—were then placed in
tanks of warm saltwater, while the doctors monitored their condition. Either while connected to this artificial placenta or
shortly after they were disconnected all the fetuses died. The
report describes the death of the largest fetus in terms that were
bound to evoke horror in anyone not inured to such events.
This fetus rested peacefully while receiving oxygenated blood
through the umbilical vein, then gasped for breath and eventually died when the artificial placenta was shut off. The researchers recorded their observations:

> For the whole 5 hours of life, the fetus did not respire,
> irregular gasping movements, twice a minute, occurred in
> the middle of the experiment but there was not proper
> respiration. Once the profusion [that is, the pumping in of
> oxygenated blood] was stopped, however, the gasping res-
> piratory efforts increased to 8 to 10 per minute. . . . After
> stopping the circuit, the heart slowed, became irregular and
> eventually stopped. . . . The fetus was quiet, making occa-
> sional stretching limb movements very like the ones re-
> ported in other human work . . . the fetus died 21 minutes
> after leaving the circuit. . . .[6]

Development of such techniques holds promise of medical
benefit and may help save the lives of undeveloped fetuses,
fetuses too young to survive despite the best efforts of doctors
and current medical technology. Thus, the American Association of Obstetricians and Gynecologists awarded this research
the Foundation Prize for important contributions to medical
science.

As fetal research grew as an important research practice, a few
thoughtful observers foresaw the possible social disruption. In
1967, in *The New York Times Magazine* James Conniff wrote
of the womb as the new frontier of science.[7] Fetal and genetic
research, he argued, would prove more important than the

exploration of space, and, drawing an analogy to another controversy over science, urged "ordinary people to call on government to prepare for the forthcoming 'revolution of the unborn' more realistically than we did for nuclear energy. . . ."[8]

In the late 1960s, many in and outside the research community expressed growing discomfort about the moral issues of research; this discomfort was, however, unfocused. This was a time when scientists and politicians were beginning to worry about the public response to these promising, yet disturbing areas of research. Dr. James Watson, the molecular geneticist and Nobel laureate, worried that unless the public addressed the moral issues embedded in biological research before they became part of routine medical practice that it would be too late. Some scientists were troubled by the tension between the press of scientific progress and the need for moral direction. "What man can do is becoming more obvious," Dr. J. Russell Elkinton told a reporter, but "What man ought to do is yet a dark enigma."[9]

In 1970, Minnesota senator Fritz Mondale, responding to those concerns, called for a national commission on medical ethics. This commission, consisting of scientists, philosophers, and citizens, would have publicly aired and debated the social and moral implications of medical research. He had expected that scientists would welcome such a commission; they didn't. Convinced that research must remain free from all outside intervention, they feared that public involvement would impede medical progress. Though research was funded by the public, the research process was, to many scientists, none of the public's business. Scrutiny should remain within the scientific community. Confronting a wall of scientific opposition, Mondale lamented, "I was disappointed and appalled by the almost unexplained fear on the part of some scientists about the public being involved."[10]

Thus public involvement in the social and moral issues of fetal research waited for the issue to become politically controversial and socially divisive. And, as we shall see, by this time the overdue debate over these issues could not be easily contained or controlled. To scientists, who resisted the national commission and feared the headaches and encumbrances of public scrutiny, the looming fetal research controversy would realize their worst nightmares. Fetal research, with its promise of discovery and therapies, eventually came to a screeching halt, and researchers who thought of themselves as contributing to the noble cause of helping unborn babies were branded by their critics as amoral, if not "mad scientists."

Foreshocks of the American controversy over fetal research were first felt in England in the early 1970s. In a powerful and grisly speech before Parliament, Norman St. John-Stevens, member of Parliament, charged scientists with profiting from the sale of fetal remains and denounced the transportation of fetuses from abortion clinics to research institutes. In response, Parliament appointed an advisory group to propose regulations. Under the leadership of Sir John Peel, a fellow of the Royal College of Obstetrics and Gynecology, the commission addressed questions about the status of the fetus and the requirements for consent for the use of the fetus and fetal remains in research.

The Peel Commission report, issued in May 1972, concluded that a planned abortion should in no way change the legal and medical protection afforded a fetus.[11] Research that would not be done on a fetus expected to go full term should not be done on a fetus scheduled for abortion: the soon-to-be-aborted fetus should not become a lab animal, according to the commission.

Its report did, however, conclude that fetal research was an essential and, if following a set of rules, an ethical form of biomedical research. The rules were that: (1) researchers must have no part in the decision on the fetus's eligibility for experimentation—someone or some group not directly involved in the research must determine eligibility, (2) the proposed research must be essential to science, and (3) any money exchanged for the procurement of fetuses and fetal tissue must cover only the costs; no one should financially gain from the sale of aborted fetuses. In addition, the report described fetuses as a new class of human subjects requiring new restrictions on acceptable research.

The Peel Commission concluded that research must consider all fetuses more than twenty weeks gestational age as potentially viable, and, in their view, viable fetuses could only be used in therapeutic research; that is, research to save or improve that fetus's life. Under the commission guidelines, nontherapeutic research was permitted on fetuses younger than twenty weeks gestational age and weighing less than 300 grams. Although such fetuses may be alive, none can sustain life outside the womb for more than fleeting moments despite the best efforts of medical science; they are considered nonviable. In such cases, the mother's consent was considered by the commission members to be necessary and sufficient for her fetus to become involved. The Peel Commission took a conspicuously cautious stance: not only were their criteria for viability conservative, but their arguments gave greater weight to the individual fetus's rights than to the scientific merit of the research.

The British discussion of fetal research was less strident than the later American controversy, but the Peel Commission report failed to resolve certain issues. For example, the working definition of viability acknowledges the medical fact that the lives of fetuses less than twenty weeks cannot be sustained, but critics asked how long a fetus must live outside the womb to be considered alive. Is life measured in days or minutes? The question of money that would later haunt fetal tissue transplantation research was also at issue: When reimbursing expenses what can be legitimately charged? Should abortion clinics be repaid for its general operating expenses and pregnant women reimbursed for prenatal care? Would this open the door to financial incentives for abortion? The Peel Commission did not resolve these controversial issues, but nonetheless it did settle the dispute in Britain and influenced later efforts to resolve the controversy in the U.S.

The troubling social and moral questions at the center of the fetal research controversy are the same in both Britain and the

U.S., yet only in America did these questions explode into rancorous conflict. For in 1973 organized antiabortion groups began to view fetal research as an issue that served their broader political strategies and goals.

The British controversy and the work of the Peel Commission were barely noticed in the U.S. They never made headlines or the nightly news, they were not commented on in Congress or the White House, but they did arouse the interest of officials at the National Institutes of Health (NIH), who knew of the growing importance of fetal research to medicine and who worried about the potential for conflict. In response, they set up a panel of scientists to make sure that NIH-supported fetal studies met ethical standards.

The panel, comprised primarily of university-based researchers, addressed many of the issues discussed by the Peel Commission, such as the definition of viability and the different rules for research on fetuses at different developmental levels. However, unlike their British counterparts, they began from a narrowly pro-research premise, basing their discussions and conclusions on the belief that fetal research was too important to limit. Thus their purpose was to define procedures to assure that fetal research of all kinds would continue.

The NIH study panel issued its report in September 1971. They recommended that researchers should pay greater attention to the mother's consent to research on an aborted fetus, but insisted that all forms of fetal research are morally acceptable and scientifically important. The report aired some of the potentially controversial issues but did not suggest any new restrictions. The panel strongly encouraged NIH to continue funding fetal research and concluded that "Planned scientific studies of the human fetus must be encouraged if the outlook for maternal and fetal patients is to be improved. Acceptable formats for the conduct of . . . carefully safeguarded, well controlled investigations *must be found*" (emphasis added).[12]

Away from the glare of public attention, then, between 1972

and 1973, NIH and Health, Education, and Welfare (HEW)[13] officials quietly debated several draft guidelines for fetal research that were based in part on the study panel's recommendations. Near the end of their deliberations, draft guidelines were published in the medical newsletter *OB-GYN News,* where they aroused little comment and no controversy. NIH's thinking on this matter closely corresponded to the views of most physicians and medical researchers: fetal research was important and ethical even if researchers needed to be more careful about obtaining informed consent from the mother.

Their expectations were to change dramatically with the 1973 Supreme Court decision, *Roe* v. *Wade,* supporting a woman's right to choose abortion. Research that had proceeded in the quiet of the laboratory, insulated from the scrutiny of those outside the scientific community, would soon be tossed in the storm of moral politics.

At the same time that fetal research was growing in importance and becoming more common, attitudes in the U.S. about abortion were changing. Prior to 1960 abortion was a "whisper-word." Although abortions became more common and more acceptable in the 1950s, they were still not discussed "in polite company or in public."[14] By 1970, abortion was no longer taboo; it was discussed more openly, and women wanting abortions no longer were forced to go abroad or find back-alley abortionists.

A shift in medical practice presaged the greater public acceptance of abortion. Through most of the twentieth century, standard medical practice permitted abortion only to save the life of the mother.[15] By 1950, however, medical texts instructed doctors to perform therapeutic abortions "for the purpose of saving the life of the mother, including her mental health or sanity. . . ."[16] Protecting the mother's mental health was interpreted by many physicians to allow the termination of unwanted pregnancies.

During this period abortions were increasingly performed in hospitals and clinics rather than in doctor's offices. This greatly increased the safety of abortion but at the same time made it more visible; abortion could no longer remain a secret between a woman and her doctor. By 1971, two years before the Supreme Court declared restrictive state abortion laws unconstitutional, as many as 600,000 legal abortions were performed in this country each year.[17] In the 1970s and 1980s, the prevalence of abortion remained relatively constant; thus, the change in the acceptance and frequency of abortion preceded the Supreme Court decision. The Supreme Court merely ratified a change that had already occurred in practice.

On January 22, 1973, U.S. Supreme Court justices decided in *Roe* v. *Wade,* by a seven-to-two vote, that the Texas anti-abortion law was unconstitutional.[18] Justice Harry Blackmun's majority opinion (Justices Byron White and William Rehnquist dissented) outlined the limits to state authority over a woman's decision to have an abortion. States were not allowed to limit abortions performed in the first or second trimester, except to require appropriate medical care. States retained the authority to outlaw abortion only after the fetus had attained viability near the end of the second trimester. In the third trimester, *Roe* v. *Wade* permitted individual states to limit a woman's legal right to choose an abortion, except in the case when the mother's life and health were placed at risk by continuing the pregnancy.

The *Roe* v. *Wade* decision rested on two pillars: the status of the fetus and the right to decide the fate of the fetus, issues that haunt the fetal research controversy. The opinion, based on reasoning similar to that of the Peel Commission, determined that at the point of viability the state asserts a compelling interest in the fetus. A viable fetus is a legal person, whereas a nonviable fetus does not have legal rights separate from the mother. Like the Peel Commission, the Court also decided that prior to the moment of viability and legal personhood the mother has the right to decide the fate of the fetus. In the Court decision, however, this right is based on the right to privacy, not the importance of informed consent. Decisions about whether or not to terminate an early pregnancy, the Court majority asserted, should remain in the "zone of privacy" where the state cannot enter without threatening liberty.

The influence of *Roe* v. *Wade* was not, however, limited to expanding legal access to abortion. Celeste Condit writes, "The revolutionary importance of the Court's decision rested . . . in its character as a national symbolic act. The *Roe* v. *Wade* case officially legitimated a new set of shared meanings which had been argued into place in the decade before the Court decision."[19] These shared meanings did not, however, represent a national consensus; rather they defined one side, what would later be called the "pro-choice" side, of the issue that since 1973 has split the nation.

By giving constitutional legitimacy to a woman's decision to have an abortion, *Roe* v. *Wade* solidified the antiabortion or Right-to-Life movement. Their loss in the Supreme Court began their search for new tactics and fresh battlegrounds to express their antiabortion views. The attention of the Right-to-Life movement shifted from the courts to the legislatures, where, among other tactics, they tried unsuccessfully to overturn *Roe* by amending the Constitution. Antiabortion activists also worked to elect sympathetic lawmakers at all levels of government.

In the years that followed *Roe* v. *Wade*, activists transformed antiabortion views from a minor electoral issue to a political absolute: as the power of the antiabortion movement grew, strong Right-to-Life stands were required of anyone seeking conservative support for either elective or appointed office. The anitabortion movement built their political influence by erasing any middle ground; regardless of their views on other issues, antiabortion groups either supported or denounced candidates for government office on this basis alone. The absolutist strategy of single-issue moral politics proved highly successful.[20]

The antiabortion movement deliberately split the nation and government institutions into pro- and antiabortion sides, and fetal research was an obvious foil. Though never a primary target of the antiabortion movement, it was seized upon as a political issue almost immediately after the 1973 *Roe* v. *Wade* decision.[21] Fetal research became a small skirmish in the larger battle over abortion; a battle, like all political battles, fought as much over symbols and images as substance. Elected officials found themselves pressured into voting for bans on fetal research despite their generally pro-research orientation because the antiabortion movement demanded absolute adherence to its views.

During this early period, the fetal research controversy was unpredictable and marked by unexpected court actions and public protests. On April 10, 1973, the front page of the *Washington Post* carried the story, "Live-Fetus Research Debated."[22] What had been discussed only among medical scientists was now headline news. The story recounted the year-old conclusions of the NIH study panel that had recommended continued support for all fetal research—the *Post* story suggested that they had become "NIH policy"—and described the artificial placenta research on living fetuses.

The status of these guidelines was confused, however. By 1973, the federal government was reconsidering all medical research guidelines in light of the public outcry against egregious violations of medical ethics in the Tuskegee Syphilis Study.[23] In July 1972, the Associated Press broke the story that for forty years the Public Health Service (PHS) had been studying the effects of untreated syphilis on indigent African American men living in Macon County, Alabama, an impoverished county of worn-out cotton farms and sharecropper shacks. What shocked the nation still in turmoil over the Civil Rights movement was that these black men were denied treatment in order to preserve the integrity of the research. Looking back from the 1970s, the research was not only ill conceived and unethical but racist as well.

The men recruited for study by the PHS were poor and mostly illiterate. All had advanced cases of syphilis. They were given free rides to and from the clinic, free physical exams, free treatment for minor ailments, hot meals on exam days, and a $50 guaranteed burial benefit paid to survivors. For many participants, this burial benefit, which was increased slightly as the study progressed, was their only legacy. The study did not involve experiments with new treatments nor better ways to manage the disease; its purpose was simply to document the progression of the disease by routine physical exams and autopsies. The study was well known among scientists interested in this area of research—numerous reports appeared in medical journals and results were openly discussed at professional conferences—but the general public did not learn of the study until it became controversial in 1972.

When the Tuskegee Study began in 1932, the cause and progression of syphilis were well known. In 1907, doctors could diagnose early syphilis with the Wassermann test, and in 1910 the first effective treatment was developed using salvarsan, a preparation of mercury and organic arsenic. The cure, a precursor to modern chemotherapy, required repeated, lengthy, often painful, and sometimes fatal doses of these toxic drugs; the treatment was often worse than the disease. In the 1930s, doctors could reasonably and compassionately argue the potential harm of the salvarsan treatment was greater than the potential benefit for advanced cases, such as those recruited in the Tuskegee Study. By 1940, however, the discovery of penicillin provided a painless and reliable cure. Nonetheless, these poor, sick men were denied treatment to continue the research for another thirty years.

In addition to the timing of this controversy, the Tuskegee Study has several implications for fetal research. Although some in the medical community continued to argue for the scientific value of the research, once the study became controversial attention focused on the moral, not the scientific, issues involved. The public was stunned by the ethical oversights of the doctors, nurses, and public health officials who focused narrowly on the research and failed to see the broader issues involved. The editors of the *Atlanta Constitution* wrote, "Sometimes, with the best of intentions, scientists and public officials and others involved in working for the benefit of us all . . . concentrate so totally on plans and programs, experiments, statistics—on abstractions—that people become objects, symbols on paper, figures in a mathematical formula, or impersonal 'subjects' in a scientific study." Anticipating complaints soon to be charged against fetal researchers, the Tuskegee scientists, according to these editors, suffered from "a moral astigmatism."[24]

The controversy over the Tuskegee Study was fundamentally different from the emerging controversy over fetal research, however. No one argued that the ethical lapses in the Tuskegee Study were justified or acceptable; it is obviously wrong to withhold an effective cure from patients, even consenting patients, merely to further scientific knowledge. But as we shall see, the ethical issues surrounding fetal research are not nearly so clear, and many argue that fetal research is moral, as well as scientifically important. Nonetheless the publicity over the Tuskegee Study forced NIH to reconsider all research procedures that included humans—including research on the fetus.

The *Post*'s disclosures of the fetal research guidelines brought national news coverage, clarifications and denials by NIH officials, and a demonstration at the NIH offices calling for a total ban on fetal research.[25] The protest, the first public demonstration ever held at NIH, was small and, by the standards of later antiabortion rallies, gentle; it resembled a high school assembly more than a protest.[26] Approximately 200 Roman Catholic high school students gathered in front of NIH. Among the protesters was a seventeen-year-old Maria Shriver, the niece of Senator Edward Kennedy, who spoke for the demonstrators. In a display of openness, NIH officials invited the protesters into an auditorium for questions and answers.

During the session, Charles Lowe, the scientific director of the National Institute for Child Health and Human Development, insisted that they had no plans to continue live-fetus research. He told the students that the advisory groups were made up of university scientists who "can say anything they want, but policy is made by NIH."[27] He insisted, nonetheless, that research on dead fetusus and fetal tissue must continue. However, the event raised more questions than it answered. Despite Lowe's assertions and the relatively few live-fetus studies, this research became a powerful symbol of scientific indifference, if not immorality, and so fetal research became a means to demonstrate the moral corrosiveness of abortion.

The 1973 protest over fetal research was short-lived, but by establishing the association of fetal research and abortion, it changed the dynamics of this conflict. Well after press coverage waned, Right-to-Life groups argued for bans and restraints on fetal research in their all-out campaign against abortion.

In addition, this first public controversy over fetal research anticipated the polarized definitions of the fetus that make compromise and solutions so elusive. Dr. Kirt Hirshorn of New York's Mount Sinai Hospital told reporters: "I don't think [fetal research on a nonviable fetus is] unethical. It's not possible to make the fetus into a child, therefore we can consider it nothing more than a piece of tissue." John Cardinal Krol, on the other hand, defines the irreconcilable premise of the opposition: "If there is a more unspeakable crime than abortion itself, it is using the victims of abortion as living human guinea pigs."[28]

This initial protest over fetal research began a twenty-year controversy that pitted our desire for medical progress against our doubts about its moral costs. Whether for or against the research, we all crave safer and better treatments for fetal diseases and abnormalities and more complete knowledge of fetal development. But, as this first protest made clear, many, especially antiabortionists, are troubled by the involvement of fetuses in the research necessary to produce this new knowledge. The issues that make fetal research so controversial are, therefore, embedded in the research itself.

2 Learning about the Fetus

The History of Our Understanding of the

Fetus and the Methods of Modern Fetal

Research

Human biological life exists in two distinct stages, pre- and postnatal, and in two distinct realms, in and outside the womb. All the changes of postnatal life—from infancy through adolescence, adulthood, and old age—pale in comparison to the changes made during the nine months of fetal life. In these months, the fetus evolves from a single cell one-tenth of a millimeter in diameter to a newborn with all the organs and systems of an adult.

In the past, we learned about the fetus indirectly through observing changes in pregnant women and examining the remains of miscarriages and stillbirths. These gave only faint clues to fetal life and development, and the most basic understanding of the fetus eluded us for centuries. Much of our knowledge of human development was inferred from observing, dissecting, and experimenting with other animals. Speculation by ancient Greeks was transmitted by Arab philosopher-physicians to medieval Christendom and to the modern world.[1] Aristotle, perhaps the first embryologist, carefully watched and recorded the day-by-day development of chicks in eggs; research that is still repeated in school biology labs around the world. But careful observation of other animals can prove misleading when applied to humans. Extrapolating from Aristotle, sixteenth-century European drawings showed the human embryo developing much like a bird in an egg (see Figure 2-1).

The invisible process of fertilization also defied explanation. The patriarchal ancient Greeks thought that semen carried the new life with the female egg supplying only nourishment. The early history of embryology was dominated by a debate over preformation. One school of thought, the "epigenesists," considered the fertilized egg as a new creation, while the preformationists described development as an unfolding of what already existed. Pushing this argument to its logical conclusion, preformationists reasoned that all future generations were held, like Chinese boxes, in the sex cells of all previous generations: inside the germ cells of the current generation were the preformed germs of the next generation, which, in turn, held the germs of the third generation, and so on through the ages. They argued that Eve held all the future generations in her ovaries and that human life would end when her supply was depleted. To ridicule this view, the physicist Nicolaus Harsocker (1656–1725) calculated the number of rabbits born since the beginning of time to demonstrate that the first rabbit could not possibly contain so many preformed rabbits.[2] Nonetheless, the preformation view persisted well into the eighteenth century; indeed, even today those who argue that genes determine individual characteristics reflect a contemporary version of the preformation doctrine.

After the discovery of spermatozoa in 1677, scientists in the early 1700s, whose observations were guided by their preformation beliefs, insisted that they could see with their microscopes tiny adults of different species with arms, legs, and heads in each sperm.[3] Some claimed to be able to distinguish donkey from horse sperm based on the length of the ears of the tiny encased animal. A group called "animalculists" or "spermists"

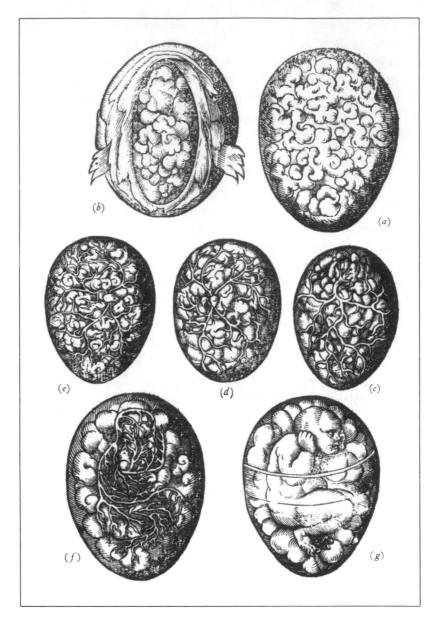

FIG. 2-1. *Egglike Embryo, from Jacob Rueff, "De Conceptu et Generatione Hominis," 1554*

Reprinted by permission from Joseph Needham, *A History of Embryology,* 2nd edition (Cambridge, England: Cambridge University Press, 1959), 113. From the collection of the Clendening History of Medicine Library, The University of Kansas Medical Center.

believed that each human sperm contained a miniature person, who raced against all others to reach the egg. They described the egg as empty and fitted with a trapdoor. The fastest sperm opened the door and climbed inside, locking the door to prevent anyone else from sharing the egg. Others, "ovists," insisted that the egg contained the germ of life with the sperm merely instigating the process of development.

Those rejecting the preformation view also shared beliefs that modern science has discredited. Many early scientists, including Aristotle, believed in the spontaneous generation of new life or parthenogenesis. Jan Baptist van Helmut (1577–1644), for example, described how fermenting wheat produced mice.

> [I]f soiled linen be pressed into the mouth of a bottle in which there is wheat, within a few days (say twenty-one) ferment drawn from the garment and changed by the odor of the grains transmutes the wheat, encrusted with its skin, into mice. . . . And it is even more remarkable that the mice which come from grain and soiled linen are by no means small or suckling, tiny or abortive, but they spring forth completely formed.[4]

Although by the nineteenth century the spontaneous generation of higher animals such as mice had long been disproved, it was not until the 1870s, when Louis Pasteur (1822–1895) showed that microorganisms and unsterile containers explained the spontaneous generation of lower forms of life, that these ideas were fully repudiated.

In the late 1600s, Dutch scientist Antonie van Leeuwenhoek (1632–1723) was the first to observe individual human sperm in a microscope. He wrote a friend of his studies:

> I had divers times examined the same matter (human semen) from a healthy man (not from a sick man, nor spoiled by keeping for a long time, and not liquified after the lapse of some minutes, but immediately after ejaculation, before six beats of the pulse had intervened): and I have seen so great a number of living creatures in it. . . .[5]

Leeuwenhoek also searched, but in vain, for the mammalian egg. He mated rabbits and killed them from six hours to six days after coitus, looking for ova in the tubes and uterus without success. The eggs of mammals are much larger than sperm—they are visible as a tiny speck to the unaided eye—but they are much more difficult to locate. Leeuwenhoek may have actually found the rabbit ova, but because he was looking for a much larger cell, he did not identify it as such. In 1828, Karl Ernst von Baer (1792–1876) was the first to identify the egg of a mammal, and Wilhelm Hertwig (1849–1922) first observed fertilization in the transparent eggs of sea urchins in 1875.

Another problem that troubled scientists for centuries was the food supply for the fetus. Making analogies to birds and plants, some early scientists postulated that the egg fed the human fetus, but the obvious inadequacy of the tiny, and at that time unseen, egg as a food source led early scientists to wonder if the fetus drank amniotic fluid. In 1677, Marguerite du Tertre, an early woman scientist, boiled amniotic fluid until it left a small amount of nonnutritious residue, ruling out this food source.[6] A leading biologist of his day, Johann von Döllinger (1770–1841), described the early embryo as a ruminant grazing on the chorion and placenta for food.[7]

The most prominent theory of fetal nutrition was based on the observation that menstrual blood ceases during pregnancy. Dating back to Hippocratic writing around 460 B.C., many believed that menstrual blood fed the developing fetus. For example, John Freind calculated in the early eighteenth century the weight of menstrual blood which, he believed, would have been produced during nine months of pregnancy. Since the weight of blood, according to his incorrect calculations, was greater than the average birth weight, he concluded that the diverted menstrual blood could provide more than enough food for the growing fetus.[8] William Harvey (1578–1657), who first described the circulation system, believed that the placenta secreted uterine milk which fed the fetus.[9]

Medieval and Renaissance scientists also wondered how the fetus could breathe submerged inside the womb. In 1659, one physician reasoned that the fetus breathed from a bubble of air at the top of the womb.[10] Until William Harvey demonstrated in the mid-seventeenth century that maternal and fetal blood vessels were separate, most physicians, dating back to ancient Rome, believed that the mother's blood vessels ran through the placenta and directly supplied the fetus with maternal blood, as if the fetus were just another of the mother's organs (see Figure 2-2). Defining the fetus as maternal tissue still dominates current medical and legal treatment of the early fetus, a topic discussed in Chapter 5. Before Harvey, many learned treatises described how the fetal and maternal blood vessels separated and closed off during labor to prevent massive bleeding at birth.[11]

Much of the early knowledge of fetal development, especially the later stages of fetal development, came from autopsies of pregnant women. In 1490, Leonardo da Vinci's accurate and beautiful drawings of a human fetus in the womb represent considerable understanding of fetal development and maternal organs, even though the sketches inaccurately depict the placenta because of his likely reliance on sheep for models (see Figure 2-3). Human maternal organs such as the placenta differ from those of even our nearest primate relatives. Perhaps even more remarkable are Jan van Rymsdyk's drawings of the fetus and uterus published in William Hunter's 1774 illustrated book, *The Anatomy of the Human Gravid Uterus* (see Figure 2-4). These plates are drawn with almost photographic accuracy, as Hunter stated, "Every part is represented just as it is found; not so much as one joint of a finger has been moved. . . ."[12]

By 1800 medical science began to understand the basic outlines of fetal development and the roles of maternal organs, such as the placenta. Although written more poetically than current medical texts, a few excerpts from the 1819 *London Medical Dictionary* illustrate some knowledge of the structural changes that occur during fetal development.

> The foetus is, for a time, invisible; and when at first seen, resembles . . . a tadpole, with a rounded head, from which a tail projects. This tail does not consist of what are after-

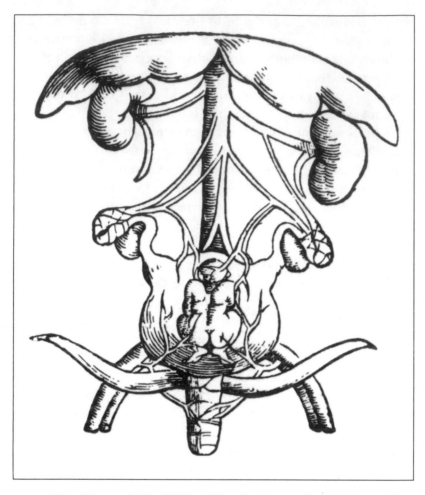

FIG. 2-2. *Maternal Blood Veins Directly Connected to the Fetus, from Walther Ryff,* Anthomia, *1541*

Reprinted by permission from Thomas Laqueur, *Making Sex: Body and Gender from the Greeks to Freud* (Cambridge, MA: Harvard University Press, 1990), 89. From the collection of the Clendening History of Medicine Library, The University of Kansas Medical Center.

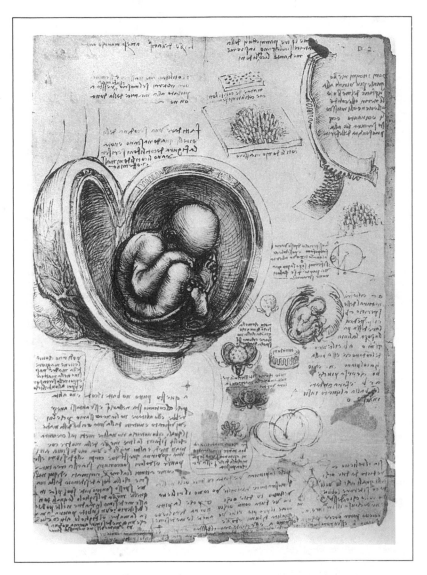

FIG. 2-3. *Leonardo da Vinci Drawing of a Human Fetus in the Womb,*
from Leonardo da Vinci's Anatomical Notebooks, *ca.* A.D. *1490*

Reprinted by permission from Royal Collection Enterprises, Photographic Services, Windsor Castle.

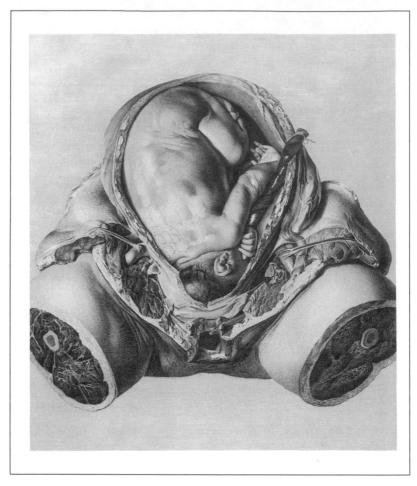

FIG. 2-4. *Jan van Rymsdyk Drawing of a Fetus in the Womb, from William Hunter,* Anatomy of the Human Gravid Uterus, *1774*

Reprinted by permission from Ove Hagelin, *The Byrth of Mankynd Otherwyse Named the Womans Booke: Embryology, Obstetrics, Gynaecology Through Four Centuries, An Illustrated and Annotated Catalogue of Rare Books in the Library of the Swedish Society of Medicine* (Stockholm: Svenska Läkaresällskapet, 1990), 129. From the collection of the Clendening History of Medicine Library, The University of Kansas Medical Center.

wards the inferior extremities, for these only appear to sprout after some months. . . .

When we can perceive any addition, we find a very minute moving point, somewhat below the head, which expands into a heart, at first conveying an almost colourless fluid, and afterwards red blood. . . .

A foetus of four weeks is near the size of a common fly; soft, mucilaginous; its bowels covered by a transparent membrane. At six weeks, it is of a somewhat firmer consistency, nearly the size of a small bee; the extremities then begin to sprout out, at three months its shape is tolerably distinct, and it is about three inches long.[13]

Many of these historical explanations and observations—sperm entering the egg through a trapdoor, a fetus breathing from a bubble, comparing its size to a bee—are quaint by modern scientific standards, but they show the emerging understanding of fetal development while underscoring the difficulty of studying the fetus. The 1800s marked major strides toward our understanding of embryology and the processes of development and differentiation, but most of the major advances still came from the biological studies of plants, insects, and nonhuman animals. For example, Louis Agassiz's major work on embryology published in 1849 does not even mention the human embryo.[14]

By the 1940s, hormonal pregnancy tests could establish the existence of a fetus, and doctors could X-ray its skeleton and hear its heartbeat. The techniques of fetal research and prenatal care had changed little from early centuries, however. Not until the 1960s did the new approaches to fetal research significantly expand our understanding of human fetal development so as to revolutionize prenatal care.

Contemporary scientists study fetuses and fetal tissue for many reasons. Some fetal research is directed at saving the life or improving the health of a specific fetus; this research includes

clinical trials of new treatments. Other research extends our
knowledge of fetal development and the causes of birth defects
in the hope of helping future fetuses. In addition, fetal cells
and tissues are used in a wide range of drug development and
testing studies. At times fetal tissue is used in research simply
because abortion makes it plentiful and it can be easily cultured
in the lab. At other times, research depends on the unique
characteristics of fetal tissue. Contemporary fetal research em-
ploys numerous procedures: some, such as morbid anatomy,
are modern adaptations of ancient practices; others, such as
using an embryoscope used to guide fetal surgery, employ the
latest medical technology.

Fetal research can involve the whole, intact fetus or just a
few cells. Much of the interest in tissue transplants centers on
fetal nerve cells or liver islet cells that are isolated and preserved
from fetal remains. Some research examines fetuses while still
in the womb, such as the further development of genetic screening through umbilical blood sampling. Other research relies on
fetuses outside the womb. These can include such drastically
different research studies as the rudimentary examinations of
miscarried remains and efforts to sustain fetal life outside the
womb with experimental life-support systems.

Some fetuses used in research are alive or exhibit life signs,
such as heartbeat. (The meaning of fetal life and death is a
difficult issue and is discussed in Chapter 4.) Clearly research
aimed at saving or providng therapy to the fetus is done on
living fetuses in the womb who are expected to develop and be
born. Other research involves dead fetuses from miscarriages
and induced abortions. Dorothy Lehrman argues that research
performed on a living fetus is, except for its reliance on fetuses,
entirely different from fetal tissue research.[15] Nevertheless the
variations among different kinds of fetal research are often obscured by political controversy so that possible abuses in one
area of research discredit other, noncontroversial projects, and
government efforts to control and restrict some types of fetal
research can inhibit or eliminate other forms that few would
find problematic on moral grounds.

Though the categories overlap somewhat, fetal research falls into five groups: studies of fetal development, the diagnosis and repair of fetal abnormalities, pharmacology and drug safety studies, research on the fetus outside the womb, and research on fetal tissue transplantation.[16] The last category, fetal tissue transplants, represents a relatively new form of research and medical treatment, and one which raises a distinct set of issues that will be discussed in Chapter 3.

Although the basic structural changes in fetal development were well known by the early twentieth century, many of the significant details of fetal development remain a mystery today. These changes occur unseen except by the diagnostic tools of modern science—the X ray, sonogram, and embryoscope—and even these provide only partial glimpses of fetal life.

Research has expanded scientific knowledge about normal fetal development. For example, we know that by ten weeks fetuses show some coordinated movement, that early fetuses (twenty-four to twenty-six weeks) respond to sound and their eyes are light sensitive in the seventh month.[17] We know little, however, about fetal cognitive development or about the nature of fetal sensation, perception, and behavior. Child-development researchers have shown that newborns demonstrate diverse and skillful responses to their environment; for example, they recognize adult faces and speech patterns. Extending this research before birth, fetal researchers are exploring, often with the help of sonograms, the development of prenatal behavior.[18]

Prior to the development of modern fetal-imaging technology, such as the sonogram, studies of fetal development were, for the most part, limited to animal studies or autopsies of dead fetuses, some of which were obtained from abortions. Several of these research protocols evoke disturbing images. One such study examined fetal brain metabolism. When malnourished, adult brains shift from sugar to fat as their energy supply to avoid cell damage. Researchers wondered if fetal brains could do the same or if they were damaged when the blood sugar supply was low, as, for example, when the mother is diabetic. To test this, they acquired nonviable fetuses of twelve to twenty-one weeks gestational age. After the fetal heartbeat stopped, and they were therefore considered dead, the researchers quickly "isolated surgically [the fetal heads] from the other organs"; the fetal corpses were, in other words, decapitated.

Researchers then inserted catheters in the carotid arteries that feed the brain and placed the heads in the organ chamber so that they could measure how rapidly the fetal brains absorbed glucose and metabolized fats. This research addressed important questions about fetal metabolism; questions that if answered could improve prenatal care. But despite the scientific value of these studies, this research would later become a symbol of unethical, "mad" science.

The development of fetal-imaging techniques has allowed researchers to look inside the womb at a living fetus and has contributed greatly to our understanding of fetal development. Although used sparingly because of fear of damage to the fetus, X rays became common in the 1930s. They revealed the changes in fetal structure and enabled researchers to inject tracer chemicals to study fetal organs, circulation, and metabolism.

The development of ultrasound imaging in the early 1970s further enhanced the researcher's ability to observe and chart changes in fetal development. Ultrasound pictures present little or no risk to the fetus and are frequently used to produce a "live" moving video of the fetus in the womb. Ultrasonography uses high-frequency, pulsating sound waves that beam painlessly into the uterus. Tissue of various density reflect different waves back to a computer, which then assembles the waves into a cross-sectional video picture.

Ultrasound images permit bone size measurements, especially the crown-rump size, that indicate accurate gestational age, and they have added to our understanding of central nervous system, kidney, and urinary tract development. These pictures are also changing the relationship of the young fetus to parents and doctors, for they give adults observing the pictures a greater sense of the reality of the as-yet-unfelt fetus. In the

New England Journal of Medicine, John Fletcher and Mark Evans observed that parents become more attached to the early fetus after viewing ultrasound images, and they speculate that ultrasound pictures will change our cultural view of the fetus to one of greater individuality.[19]

Prenatal imaging is extending closer to the moment of conception. Dr. Rubén Quintero of Wayne State University and Dr. E. Albert Reece of Temple University are among a handful of researchers experimenting with embryoscopy.[20] The embryoscope is a thin, flexible optical device much like those used to look inside blood vessels. Although its use is highly experimental, and it is used only on women already planning to have abortions, the embryoscope allows doctors to observe embryos as young as six weeks old. Such embryos are approximately three-quarters of an inch long but have tiny toes, hands, and ears. (See Figure 2-5.)

Not only will the embryoscope allow the direct observation of early development, but doctors may, if it proves safe, use it for the early identification and surgical repair of birth defects. Dr. Quintero recently used the embryoscope to guide tiny surgical tools to save a fetus who was endangered by a malformed twin.[21] The baby, Santerras Graham, was the first baby born after such an operation, though endoscopic surgery using needle-sized holes and miniature cameras is becoming more common with adults. The embryoscope, like the sonogram, may alter our image of the early embryo; it becomes less of a biological abstraction and more of an individual when we can see it and provide it with medical care.

Fetal development, except through the windows of modern technology, proceeds hidden from sight, but problems in development are painfully visible after birth. One extra chromosome and a child is born with Down's syndrome and faces a foreshortened life of mental retardation and physical problems. Fetal alcohol syndrome, crack babies, sickle-cell disease, cystic fibrosis, and Tay-Sachs disease are but a few of the more

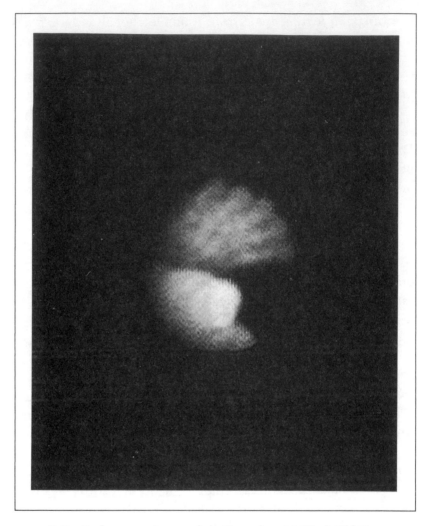

FIG. 2-5. *Embryoscope Image of the Foot of an 11-Week-Old Fetus*
Reprinted by permission from Hutzel Hospital, the Detroit Medical Center.

common environmental genetic forms of birth defects. Fetal research has contributed greatly to developing and then refining prenatal diagnostic tests.

Many birth defects lead to miscarriages and stillbirths, others to partial disability, and some, such as anencephaly—congenital absence of all or a major portion of the brain—result in near total disability and near certain death. Some, such as PKU (phenylketonuria), can be fully corrected if identified promptly. Birth defects have taught us a great deal about fetal development and the dependence of the fetus on the pregnant woman. They have also pushed medical science to develop diagnostic tools and treatments to deal with their tragic hold on postnatal life.

Fifty years ago prenatal diagnosis of birth defects was limited to examining the mother and genetic counseling. These techniques, still important today, allowed physicians to assess the possibility that something might be wrong, but these diagnoses could be confirmed or denied only after birth or miscarriage. They left the pregnant woman with the difficult choice of what to do when a doctor tells her that she has a 70 percent, or perhaps a 20 percent, chance of having a deformed child. In contrast, modern diagnostic procedures allow physicians to directly assess the health of a specific fetus.[22] Rather than concluding that the fetus has a known statistical risk for a birth defect, modern prenatal diagnosis can tell if this individual fetus is healthy or stricken.

Some prenatal diagnostic tests such as alpha-fetoprotein (AFP) screening of the mother's blood and sonograms present no risk to the fetus and are becoming standard practice. The AFP test, for example, was developed to detect defects in the developing brain and spinal cord, such as anencephaly and spina bifida. Abnormally high levels of AFP in the mother's blood indicate problems in the fetus's developing nervous system. Low levels may indicate Down's syndrome. An experimental AFP screening program in California eventually included 60 percent of pregnancies statewide.[23] Such a screening program is experimental in the sense that this test is not yet standard medical practice, but since the tests impose no risk to the fetus such research is not in itself controversial.

Other common diagnostic procedures such as amniocentesis impose some risk to the fetus.[24] During amniocentesis a long needle extracts amniotic fluid from the womb. Fetal cells are centrifuged out and cultured for chromosomal, DNA, and biochemical analysis.[25] Amniocentesis is now so routine in women over thirty-five or those with a history of genetic disorders that it is no longer considered experimental. The procedure, however, requires waiting until the fetus is sixteen weeks old before sampling fluid and three or more additional weeks to culture cells and analyze the results.

A more experimental procedure, chorionic villus sampling, allows earlier results. The chorion is the membrane that surrounds the early fetus; it develops into the placenta. Cells from the chorion contain the same fetal genetic information as provided by amniocentesis. The procedures for this diagnostic test are less well established, although studies indicate no greater risk to the fetus than amniocentesis.

Direct fetal blood sampling may be required to identify other birth defects, such as incompatibility of the mother's and fetus's blood proteins (Rh factors) and low pH levels. One promising technique involves the use of a fetoscope to guide the sampling of fetal blood. Though animal studies preceded the fetoscope's use on humans, its initial application involved unknown risks to the fetus, since small amounts of fetal bleeding can prove life-threatening. French scientists have recently developed a less risky procedure, called percutaneous umbilical blood sampling, in which physicians guided by ultrasound use a needle to sample fetal blood from the umbilical cord.

Genetic screening is also extending closer and closer to the moment of conception. For example, British doctors have tested early embryos for cystic fibrosis.[26] These embryos were fertilized in labs where researchers were able to remove a single cell from tiny embryos comprised of only four to eight cells. Genes from these single cells were then tested for the genetic disease so that the embryo that was implanted in the mother would be free of the defect. This preimplantation diagnosis allows doctors to assure would-be parents that they will not transmit a specific genetic disease.

The diagnosis of diseases of the embryo is a logical extension of in vitro fertilization; why implant genetically defective embryos? These new procedures may change the way we think about reproduction and genetic choices, however. In addition, these new procedures occur in an ethical gray area, since most doctors and investigators do not treat early embryos as human research subjects that warrant protection. As Dr. Albert Johnson of the University of Washington Medical Center told a reporter, "We really don't think that our ethical principles began to kick in until after [the embryo] stage."[27]

It is possible that in the future doctors will be able to repair the genes in early embryos. Embryos and fetuses develop rapidly, and a genetic defect quickly becomes reproduced in thousands of cells. If doctors can repair the defective genes when the embryo consists of just a few cells, it is possible to erase the genetic defect before it can harm the fetus. "This is an early glitch on the radar screen of twenty-first-century medicine," Arthur Caplan, then director of the Center for Bioethics at the University of Minnesota, commented. "The image we have today of a couple whose reproductive choices are mainly conferred by an obstetrician-gynecologist in a clinic is going to evolve into the genetic doctor peering into a microscope and sorting out embryos."[28]

Medical researchers are much closer to developing remedial procedures for fetal defects that are limited to a single organ or a specific congenital malformation.[29] For example, obstructive hydrocephalus occurs five to twenty-five times in each 10,000 births. This blockage of the fetal brain's fluid pathways leads to brain compression. The surgical insertion of a one-way shunt in the fetus's brain drains the fluid and allows normal brain development. Similar procedures are being developed to relieve urethral blockages that damage the developing kidney.

Lambs and nonhuman primates develop similar brain and kidney blockages, and these two forms of fetal surgery were extensively tested in animals before human trials. However, animal surrogates do not exist for most human genetic and metabolic disorders, and developing prenatal surgery depends on fetal experiments in the preliminary as well as final stages of development. Nevertheless, medical science is in the early stages of major advances in prenatal therapy and surgery. Glenn Griener comments:

> From the medical point of view, fetal surgery resembles organ transplantation in its early days: it seems to offer hope of effective treatment where none existed. Fetuses who were doomed to early death, or to a life of serious impairment, may now be saved from these fates.[30]

Direct treatment of the fetus not only brings promise of therapeutic interventions; it has also changed our views of the fetus. When we could not see the fetus, could not identify developing health problems, and could not treat those that we could diagnose, the fetus remained out of the public spotlight. Ironically, the technical ability to treat the fetus—a consequence of research—has further intensified controversy over the ethics of research.

Two of the most dramatic events in modern medicine, the great success of the polio vaccine and the haunting tragedy of thalidomide, indirectly involved fetal research in the development and testing of drugs, another prominent form of fetal research. The development of the Salk antipolio vaccine relied on human fetal cell cultures. Like the AIDS epidemic of today, the fear of polio, a crippling disease that sentenced many to years in the iron lung, gripped the nation during the 1930s and 1940s. "When on April 12, 1955, epidemiologists at the University of Michigan announced the results showing that the vaccine had worked, pandemonium swept the country. . . . The magic of science and money had worked."[31]

The role of fetal cells in this medical success story has become part of the mythology surrounding fetal research. Scientists often repeat the story to demonstrate the value of this research; banning fetal research, they claim, would preclude similar breakthroughs in the future.[32] But many kinds of tissues were used in the development of the polio vaccine and fetal tissue may not have been essential.[33] Nonetheless, fetal tissue cells are commonly used in developing treatments for a range of diseases. The human cell strains, with the clinical names of WI-38 and MRC-5, are derived from fetal lung cells and are essential supplies in many pharmacology labs for the development and testing of vaccines.[34]

If the polio vaccine symbolizes the successes of modern medicine, then thalidomide babies warn of its failures. Physicians are also concerned that many medications, such as antibiotics, may harm a developing fetus; and some advise avoiding all medication. "The fetus is not an innocent bystander if maternal treatment necessitates medical intervention," John Hansen and John Sladek write. "Virtually all commonly used drugs with the possible exception of insulin, heparin, dextrose, and thyroxine pass through the placenta to varying degrees."[35]

Many pharmacological studies involve tests using other animals or human fetal cells, but these may not forewarn scientists of the effects of drugs on a developing fetus. Studies of the effects of drugs on the living fetus are often retrospective, involving the examination of the fetus or infant after accidental exposure. For example, researchers studied the effects of oral contraceptives on fetuses by following the prenatal and postnatal history of children whose mothers became pregnant while using the birth-control pill. Other studies are associated with therapy, such as the use of penicillin to treat fetal syphilis. Pregnant women were also included in tests of the rubella vaccine.[36] Rubella or German measles was a leading cause of birth defects. Like many vaccines, this one involved giving the woman a mild case of rubella so that she would develop immunity. Doctors were concerned that the vaccine, like the disease, could cause birth defects if given to a pregnant woman.

In 1972 and 1973, a joint Finnish and U.S. research project examined the effects of the rubella vaccine on the developing fetus. These researchers, including one from Case Western Reserve University and another from NIH, injected the rubella vaccine into thirty-five pregnant women in Finland. These women were planning abortions and, therefore, consented to the inoculation. Laboratory studies of the fetal remains, some of them done in the U.S., documented the danger of the early vaccine on the fetus. Further refinements of the German measles vaccine has helped prevent untold thousands of birth defects, but this research, like so much fetal research, depended on planned abortion. What woman would consent to taking an unproven vaccine that could potentially damage her wanted baby?

A small number of investigations involve living fetuses in order to follow the movement of drugs, such as anesthetics given to the mother during labor, across the placenta. To increase the scientific rigor of such experiments, researchers may ask pregnant women who are planning abortions to take the drug so that the effects on the fetus can be carefully studied after the abortion.

One such study began in the early 1970s. Dr. Agnita Philipson, a Swedish physician, who was a visiting researcher at the Boston City Hospital, told her American colleague, Dr. Leon Sabath, of an observation she made while pregnant: medications she took prior to her recent pregnancy seemed less effective when she took them while pregnant. Her personal experience led her to search the medical literature only to discover how little was known about how pregnant women metabolize drugs. This conversation led to a joint research project to study the differential effects of two common antibiotics, erythromycin and clindamycin, on women who were and were not pregnant.

When Drs. Philipson and Sabath prepared their proposal for review by the hospital's ethical review board, they decided to use women planning abortion as an extra measure of safety. "As we thought about it," Dr. Sabath recalled, "we realized the safest course would be to get pregnant women who were going to have an abortion anyway. There was no reason to think that either antibiotic would be harmful to the fetus—each is widely used—but it seemed wrong to take any chance."[37]

The research was approved and the two doctors contacted a third, Dr. David Charles, who performed abortions at Boston

City Hospital. With his help, the research team found women who were planning abortion and who consented to participate in the research. As the research proceeded, the doctors also became curious about the effects of the antibiotics on the fetus. They decided to measure how readily these drugs crossed the placenta; information that could refine the treatment of fetal infections, such as fetal syphilis. The three researchers then contacted a fourth, Dr. Leonard Berman, who was a pathologist and could help them examine the fetal remains. Their findings were published in the *New England Journal of Medicine* on June 7, 1973, six months after the Supreme Court abortion ruling; a historical coincidence that would prove fateful.

A year later, Drs. Berman, Charles, Philipson, and Sabath were indicted for grave-robbing. (Dr. Philipson had returned to Sweden and avoided arrest.) In their guerilla war against abortion, Right-to-Life activists, including those in the Boston district attorney's office, looked for any means to discredit everything and everyone associated with abortion. According to the district attorney, these doctors had violated the Violation of Sepulture, or grave-robbing statute, of Massachusetts by examining the remains of the aborted fetuses without the specific permission of the mother for this aspect of their research. This long forgotten 1814 statute states:

> Whoever, not being lawfully authorized by the proper authorities, wilfully digs up, disinters, removes or conveys a human body or the remains thereof . . . shall be punished in the state prison for not more than three years or in jail for not more than two and one half years or by a fine of not more than two thousand dollars.

According to the district attorney, the aborted fetus was a human body like any other corpse and these researchers were grave-robbers, even if the "grave" was a specimen jar in a hospital lab.

After the arrests, the Boston City Hospital, a public hospital, suspended the three doctors who were still in their employ.

Although the case never came to trial and the doctors were quickly and apologetically reinstated, medical researchers were stunned by the possibility that they could be arrested for doing research approved by, even lauded by, their scientific colleagues. The editors of the *Medical Tribune* came to their defense, writing, in outrage, "This attack upon physicians openly engaged in medical research under protocols subject to the approval of a committee of peers is a major violation of humanity."[38]

After these arrests, Boston City Hospital no longer actively supported fetal research, and researchers began looking over their shoulders wondering how and when they would next be attacked. They did not have long to wait. When the prosecutors were looking for evidence in the grave-robbing case in the Boston City Hospital morgue, they found the remains of another fetus. Investigations of this fetus, later called "baby boy" in court, led to the arrest and eventual conviction of Dr. Kenneth Edelin for manslaughter. (We return to the Edelin story in Chapter 4.)

A rare form of fetal research involves experiments on the nonviable fetus that is outside the womb, the so-called fetus *ex utero*. (The term "fetus *ex utero*" is a medical oxymoron, since once a fetus is outside the womb it is no longer considered a fetus but an abortus, stillbirth, or live birth.[39]) The major developmental change at the threshold of viability is the ability of the fetus to breathe. Prior to viability the fetus has lungs and a circulation system but does not yet have the capacity to respire independently. Nonviable fetuses are, therefore, in some ways alive, demonstrating heartbeat and some nervous system activity, but current medical science cannot sustain their life. They show, however fleetingly, life signs, but cannot maintain these life signs outside the womb even with the latest advances of modern medicine. Because of this ambiguous status, research on the nonviable fetus *ex utero* proved intensely controversial.

Medical researchers use nonviable fetuses *ex utero* to measure amino acid and hemoglobin levels in the blood and to study fetal metabolism by injecting noradrenaline and tracer chemicals into the umbilical vein. In the late 1960s and early 1970s, a small number of studies, like the one discussed earlier, used these fetuses to test novel life-support systems. Later this research, like the severed fetal heads study, would be cited again and again as grotesque examples of unethical research on the dying. Images of fetal heads lined up on organ chambers and gasping fetuses floating in tanks bring to mind, as Maggie Scarf observed, "old tales of mad science [and] living beings preserved in tanks."[40] Such research symbolized to abortion opponents how the acceptance of abortion by doctors had legitimated such horrors; these studies became part of the political imagery of the antiabortion movement.

Many scientists and bioethicists were caught off guard by the emotional response such research evokes. One pro-research bioethicist, Joseph Fletcher, spoke for many scientists in his dismay at the public's gut reaction to fetal research. "Many people's belief propositions are entirely visceral, not rational— witness, for example, the repugnance some people feel at the profusion of a separated fetus head while feeling none at the profusion of its kidney."[41] But to most people outside the medical community a fetal head is fundamentally, if only symbolically, different from a fetal kidney. Medical and scientific training encourage doctors to approach questions, even ethical questions, with a colder, more rational eye than the lay public. Many simply cannot understand how this research and these issues can be so routine to scientists but so shocking to others. Consequently such research stopped after the first wave of public controversy in 1973.

3 Fetal Tissue Research

Its Uses, Benefits, and the

Inevitable Controversy That Arises

Scientists need human cells for a wide range of studies, from basic research on human genetics to developing and testing new drugs and vaccines. Biomedical and pharmaceutical labs depend on the availability of human cell cultures for the reproduction of human viruses both for the diagnosis of diseases and the production of human vaccines.[1] Scientists often use any available sources of human tissue in research; for intance, foreskins discarded after circumcisions were used in the development of the polio vaccine. To the scientist, fetal cell cultures are merely one of the better and more readily available sources of human tissue, for a small quantity of fetal cells can be easily cultured, and when cultures need to be refreshed with new cells, abortion provides an abundant supply.

First done in the 1930s, the use of fetal cell cultures has become a routine, if not widely recognized or publicized, aspect of biomedical research. Because of their special characteristics, fetal cell cultures have contributed to the understanding of the microbiology of fetal development, cell organization, and disease resistance. One current study is examining the effects of smoking on the fetus by studying the carcinogenicity of tobacco smoke on fetal cells.

Fetal cell cultures are mainly used in developing vaccines. For example, the human diploid cell strains WI-38 and MRC-5 are commonly used in vaccine development. These commercially available cell cultures, derived from fetal lung cells, are used in a wide range of research projects that require human cells. Ordering fetal cell cultures is no different than requisitioning other lab supplies, and to date this area of fetal research has been spared public controversy, though most fetal cell cultures are originally derived from aborted tissue. However, the use of these cultures in transplants is another story.

Fetal tissue transplants depend on the unique characteristics of fetal cells. Fetal tissue grows much faster than adult tissue— a few donor cells could potentially grow to replace a large number of host cells—and fetal tissue is less specialized. Developmental biologists believe that early fetal cells have the potential to become any type of adult tissue, but at the earliest stages, the embryo is too small to yield enough cells for transplantation. As the fetus grows, cells take on more and more specialized functions and reproduce others that replace their specialization. In an adult, tissue is highly specialized—muscle tissue cannot take on the work of the liver—but cells taken from fetuses, perhaps into the third trimester, retain much of their adaptability.

Fetal tissue also has a less specific immune response and is therefore less likely to be rejected when transplanted. Although some research suggests that fetal tissue transplants may elicit an immune response from the host, most researchers anticipate few problems when transplanting fetal tissue. Thus patients receiving fetal tissue transplants may be spared the lifelong regimen of antirejection medicine required after most transplants.

In adult organ transplants, the transplanted heart or kidney remains a biological outsider; these organs never become truly integrated into the host's body. Doctors do not look to fetal tissue for major organ transplants—the organs are too small and undeveloped—but fetal tissue transplants are likely to become an indistinguishable living part of the recipient.[2] Because it has a greater potential than adult tissue to actually restore the damage and to replace biochemical functions, it is an easier procedure.

As in auto repair, transplanting adult organs involves replacing defective parts: the nonworking kidney or heart is removed and a working one is installed.[3] By using fetal tissue one can, at least theoretically, transplant only a few cells or tissue fragments, which will then adapt to the host and replace the missing functions or damaged cells. In some cases, the transplantation involves little more than injecting dissociated fetal cells into the host; these cells then migrate to the appropriate site and become part of the recipient's anatomy.

In other cases, the transplantation site must be prepared and the cells or tissue fragment placed in the specific location. Two operations may be necessary to transplant tissue plugs or blocks.[4] In the first, the surgeons "pre-lesion" the site for the transplantation by making an incision. Like tilling the soil, this procedure prepares the host to accept the tissue graft by encouraging more blood vessels to appear: it creates a "vascularized" bed. The second operation involves the actual transplant of the tissue graft into the prepared site. Such transplantation is unlikely to require major surgery because the tissue is not surgically connected to the host but is placed in the appropriate spot and then, if successful, grows on its own. The challenge is to find the exact sites.

A highly experimental procedure, the long-term value of fetal tissue transplants remains to be assessed. Nonetheless, tissue grafts from fetuses to adults, especially aged adults, may become an entirely new form of medical treatment; for they promise remedies for some of the most devastating adult diseases, such as Parkinson's and Alzheimer's, that have long resisted cures. Fetal tissue transplantation may become a medical breakthrough similar to the first vaccines, and the fetus may become a pharmacopoeia supplying cells and tissues used to cure many diseases.

Fetal tissue has one additional characteristic that makes it both attractive to medical science and socially controversial: because of the frequency of abortion, fetal tissue is abundant.[5] Most abortions now occur in hospitals or clinics where tissue can be properly recovered and stored; therefore, if or when fetal tissue transplants become accepted medical procedures, the supply of tissue should not be a major problem. Because abortion provides a constant supply, recipients needing fetal tissue will not need to wait for months or years, as do those needing hearts or kidneys.

Medical science has long recognized these special properties of fetal tissue, and doctors have for years speculated on its possibilities. After reviewing a century of fetal tissue studies, one critic concluded that the often extravagant claims made for fetal tissue transplants are based more on medical folklore than solid research.[6] Nevertheless, most scientists concur with Dr. Warran Olanow's assessment that it is "very promising."[7] Fetal brain grafts in animals date back a hundred years. Over seventy years ago, Dr. Elizabeth Dunn reported that tissue from a fetal rat brain survived transplantation and showed evidence of growth and integration into the host brain.[8] Several generations of animal studies, including transplants across species, indicate that fetal tissue transplants are biologically possible. While it is not yet clear if fetal transplants will work in humans, the basic mechanism does work in other animals. Medical researchers, therefore, look to fetal tissue transplantation as a possible cure for any number of disabilities and diseases that result from the body's inability to repair itself.

Of all the forms of fetal tissue transplantation, fetal nerve grafts are the most thoroughly studied. Research with animals provides strong evidence that these grafts survive and grow. The ease and speed with which the grafts grow in the host may even present a major problem: in some primate studies, the fetal nerve tissue transplant grew too large and, like a tumor, damaged the host brain. Although most of the research involves rats and other lab animals, not humans, fetal tissue has been

successfully transplanted in nearly every area of the central
nervous system. As Hansen and Sladek suggested in *Science,*
"Virtually every region of the central nervous system, from the
olfactory neuroepethelium to the spinal cord, can be grafted
[with fetal tissue], with minimal immunological consequences."[9]

Medical researchers consider fetal tissue transplantation as a
possible cure for any number of adult degenerative nerve diseases, such as Parkinson's and Alzheimer's; it may also repair
brain and spinal cord injuries. Injury or disease that damages
adult nerves is permanent because adults cannot produce new
nerve cells. When the surviving nerves find new pathways to
old skills, as when a stroke victim relearns to walk, the effects
of brain injuries are mitigated but not eliminated. Fetal nerve
cells, in contrast to mature ones, grow and adapt to new functions, so that fetal tissue transplants may actually repair or replace the damaged nerves, thereby holding promise, however
faint, of miracle cures: the wheelchair-bound walking and the
catatonic regaining awareness.

However, it is not clear from the animal studies how fetal
tissue transplants actually restore lost nerves and nervous system
functions. The transplanted tissue may stimulate host nerves to
grow, or it may release, or encourage the host tissue to release,
the biochemical signals that permit nerve cell reproduction. The
fetal tissue transplant may also act as a replacement source, or
"local pump," for the chemical neurotransmitters that are essential to brain activities. Some researchers suggest that the fetal
tissue graft may actually restore the broken synapse circuity, in
effect rewiring the damaged brain.

Most of the research on fetal neural transplants in humans
involves Parkinson's disease patients. At this time, cures for
Alzheimer's disease or brain and spinal cord injuries remain
hopes, not empirically tested procedures. Parkinson's is a degenerative brain disease that begins with tremors in the hands
and legs and proceeds—sometimes gradually, sometimes rapidly—to near total loss of nervous system control and sometimes to rigid, near frozen muscles. Although incapacitating—
advanced cases have difficulty with such basic acts as swallow-

ing—the disease rarely diminishes mental abilities until its later stages, when Parkinson's patients often develop symptoms of Alzheimer's disease. Being so incapacitated yet aware adds to the special tragedy of Parkinson's.

Parkinson's disease afflicts a half a million Americans and many other millions worldwide, yet the cause of most cases is not known. In most instances, the brain of a Parkinson's patient has, as the disease progresses, fewer and fewer *substantia nigra* cells. As this region of the brain atrophies, it no longer produces an adequate supply of dopamine, an essential neurotransmitter. There is no cure for Parkinson's disease, but its symptoms can be alleviated and the progression of the disease slowed by the use of drugs, such as levo-deoxyphenenylalanine (L-dopa), that stimulate dopamine production. Eventually drug treatment fails because the continuing loss of brain cells makes dopamine production no longer possible.

If fetal tissue transplants can either replace or stimulate the growth of the *substantia nigra,* the cure of Parkinson's is, at least theoretically, possible.[10] At a minimum, this procedure could substitute or reduce the need for drug therapy. The first published reports of the success of fetal tissue transplants to treat Parkinson's were made in 1988. In a letter to the *New England Journal of Medicine,* Mexican doctors described two fetal tissue transplants; one using *substantia nigra* tissue and the other adrenal medullary tissue.[11] The letter describes substantial reduction in the symptoms of Parkinson's, but some scientists question the veracity of the research.[12] Similar findings were reported in Britain, however, and studies in Sweden found short-term clinical gains that diminished over time. In the U.S., medical researchers at the University of Colorado and Yale University report some success in their use of fetal tissue transplants in Parkinson's patients and in extensive experiments on animals. For example, Dr. Curt Freed and his colleagues injected fetal tissue into seven Parkinson's patients, and all showed measurable gains.[13] Brain scans from this research indicate increased activity in the regions where atrophy causes Parkinsonism.

Fetal tissue transfer experiments are problematic, however; many studies lack control groups and often rely solely on patient reports of improvements. The few studies with control groups found that patients who did not receive the treatment also reported improvements, raising doubts about studies without controls.[14] In addition, most studies have very few subjects. The Neural Transplant Program of Yale University's School of Medicine has reported clinically measurable gains, but no cure, in Parkinson's patients receiving fetal tissue transplants.[15] This research included a control group, but the findings, derived from several years of work, were based on just eight patients, four in the treatment and four in the control group.[16] One of the patients in the treatment group died four months after receiving the transplant, and as it turned out an autopsy revealed that he did not have Parkinson's but another disease with similar symptoms.

With such small numbers of patients in clinical trials, cautious researchers are loath to overstate the value of fetal tissue transplants. As Yale's Dr. Redman suggests, the symptoms of Parkinson's can vary from day to day: "One of the classic stories about Parkinson's disease is that the patient can be in a wheelchair for years; then their house catches fire and they jump up out of the wheelchair and run for the door."[17]

Although fetal neural tissue research has received the most attention, doctors are exploring other forms of fetal tissue transplants. The only accepted use of this novel form of medicine involves the transplantation of fetal thymus cells to treat DiGeorge's syndrome (also called congenital thymic hypoplasia). With this rare and devastating birth defect, a baby is born without a working thymus and with little or no immune suppression. Babies born with DiGeorge's often have deformed faces and abnormal hearts and kidneys in addition to their lack of immunity.

DiGeorge's syndrome is so rare that no one knows the actual number of incidents. Mild cases can be treated with surgery and medication, but for extreme cases, fetal thymus transplants offer the only real hope of cure. Still, the small number of transplants done each year and the limited success of the operation raise doubts about the value of transplanting fetal thymus cells. One review found only 31 percent of babies having this transplant survived for an extended period of time after the operation.[18] Severe cases of DiGeorge's syndrome nearly always lead to rapid death; therefore, a one-third survival rate is a marked improvement in the treatment, if not a cure, of this rare disease.

The success, however limited, of fetal tissue transplants in restoring the immune system for DiGeorge's syndrome babies gives some hope for finding cures for other congenital immune system problems. For example, some children are born with a genetic defect that leaves them unable to produce any lymphocytes, the white blood cells that fight disease. This extremely rare disorder is called Severe Combined Immune Deficiency syndrome, or SCIDs. Children without working immune systems are either forced to live in a completely sterile environment, such as the "boy in the bubble," or usually die of infection before their first birthday, because at this time the only treatment of SCIDs is a bone-marrow transplant from a closely matched donor. Such donors are not available for well over half of the patients, and for this reason researchers are experimenting with fetal liver and thymus transplants. They report some success; although only a few of the patients are cured, the transplants do appear to survive and function in the host. But with refined procedures these transplants may offer an alternative in the treatment of SCIDs.[19]

Fetal transplant techniques also hold some promise in AIDS research. One of the barriers to AIDS research is finding an inexpensive animal model of the disease. Until researchers can create lab animals that mimic the human disease, they are forced to leap quickly from studies of cells to human trials. Some researchers are now trying to give AIDS to mice and rats by first transplanting the human immune system into the immune-deficient rodents, a process that relies on human fetal liver and thymus transplants. Researchers have created a lab mouse without an immune system, the hu-SCID mouse, that is used to test HIV vaccines.[20] If, in addition, they can transplant a human immune system into these lab mice, then they can give them AIDS and use them in studies of both the causes and cures for the disease.

It is also possible, although highly speculative, that fetal tissue transplants could, at least temporarily, bolster or restore the immune system of patients with AIDS. Few doctors are willing to speculate that fetal tissue transplants may one day help end this pandemic, but the partial success with other immune diseases does raise the possibility.

Fetal liver transplants may, in addition, help cure a wide range of blood diseases, such as leukemia and radiation sickness. For example, in 1986, after the Chernobyl nuclear power plant explosion, Dr. Robert Gale tried, as a last resort, to transplant fetal liver cells to regenerate the bone marrow in radiation victims. A very small number of cells located in the bone marrow, called stem cells, produce the blood supply in healthy adults. These cells are destroyed or weakened by radiation. In human fetuses, the liver, not the bone marrow, is the major producer of blood cells, and Dr. Gale hoped that fetal liver transplants could jump-start the stalled blood production of the radiation victims. Although earlier experiments with sheep gave reason for hope, all of the patients died from radiation burns before the success of the transplants could be measured.[21]

This heroic effort to save radiation victims underscores one of the major difficulties in assessing the value of fetal tissue transplants. Since these transplants are considered highly experimental, they are tried only as a last resort with patients with no hope of survival using standard medical practices. The chance of success is so remote, given the status of the patient, that failure may not indicate the potential of the operation; death does not necessarily mean that the treatment failed. In such experimental procedures, doctors do not use survival or cure as the only measure of success; they look to see if the transplants took hold and began to function. Often autopsies reveal more about experimental treatments than does the fate of the patient.

Finally, medical researchers have looked to fetal tissue transplants for a cure for diabetes. Using fetal tissue to treat diabetes was first suggested in 1903 and first attempted in Italy in 1928. Doctors in the U.S. tried the operation in 1939.[22] None of these early experiments showed any signs of success. But recently, fetal pancreas transplants have reversed drug-induced diabetes in animals. Easily cultured in the lab, a few starter cells, called islet cells, can engender large quantities of fetal pancreas cells.

Fetal pancreas transplants have also been used in about 600 diabetic humans, but there is no clear evidence that the procedure works. Most of the operations were done in the Soviet Union and China, and the published reports often lack the background information needed to assess their value. Thirty-eight patients have received various forms of fetal pancreatic transplants in the U.S. These operations have stimulated little, if any, secretion of insulin, an especially discouraging result given the success of the operation in animals and the routine use of adult kidney transplants for severe cases.

Critics of fetal tissue transplantation look at this research record and claim that the potential benefits of these transplants are overstated: Peter McCullagh says, "The relevance of the history of research on foetal tissue transplantation for medical practice . . . lies not in an endowment of hard, reproducible data but in one of impressions, often poorly founded."[23] He also insists that the value of fetal tissue transplants, like all medical procedures, must be evaluated not in the absolute but in relation to other established procedures or lines of research. In this regard, McCullagh, among others, believes that other cures for Parkinson's, leukemia, or diabetes have greater potential.

Another critic, Dr. Jonathan Pincus, chairman of the neurology department of Georgetown University, argued, in testimony before Congress, that investigating the use of fetal nerve transplants as a cure for Parkinson's was misguided and possibly abusive. In his view, the only potential benefit would be to reduce the need to give Parkinson's sufferers L-dopa: if patients do not respond to medical treatment, then there is no hope that they will respond to the transplant, since the promise of transplants is that they will stimulate dopamine production.

According to Pincus, the risk and discomfort to the patient of surgery and the remote chance of any clinical gain should preclude the experimental operation. He denounced doctors for putting their career interest in finding new treatments over the care of their patients. He testified:

> Mexican neurosurgeons recently pioneered adrenal cell transplants in Parkinson's disease with glowing reports of success reported in the *New England Journal of Medicine.* American surgeons hurried to catch up. The conclusion now is that it doesn't work. They beat us to the punch, but what was the punch? The punch was that several hundred old people have been subjected to adrenalectomies and craniotomies with no benefit and at considerable risk to them.[24]

Supporters of fetal tissue transplants acknowledge the limits of the research and recognize as disadvantages the inadequate samples, the lack of control groups, and the incomplete reporting. There are many reasons to be skeptical; nevertheless, success in animal research strongly supports the promise of fetal tissue transplantation. However fantastic the idea of using fetal tissue to restore lost brain or organ functions appears to be, medical researchers are loath to leave its potential unexplored.

For those outside the medical community, these scientific reservations are less important than concerns about the procurement and supply of fetal tissue. When scientists need fetal cells for biomedical research, they commonly order them from medical supply companies. Some labs may develop their own fetal cell cultures, but this is not the norm. Researchers using these catalog-ordered cultures know little, if anything, about the original source for the cells; they are a standardized product.

Providing tissue for transplantation experiments is much less routine. When physicians and researchers need fetal tissue for research or therapy, they develop private relationships with hospitals or clinics performing abortions. The nature of the relationship between the researcher and the tissue provider is not well known and varies markedly from place to place. There is little standardization in the collection and distribution of fetal tissue; the procurement of human fetal tissue is, perhaps, the "least structured and organized" of all the forms of tissue and organ donation.[25] "This sleazy, scummy world of fetal tissue procurement," bioethicist Arthur Caplan told a reporter, "cries out for Federal regulation."[26]

The lack of standardized procedures for collecting and transferring fetal tissue is, in part, a result of the abortion controversy. Anything associated with abortion is potentially explosive, and researchers would prefer to keep their uses of fetal remains out of the public spotlight. Controversy has forced procurement to go underground, where it is difficult to describe, much less regulate.

The secrecy surrounding the procurement of fetal tissue, however, affects research progress. An NIH study found that because researchers kept basic information about the source and status of the fetal tissue "confidential," few published reports provide details about the fetal tissue used in the research. When researchers do not include basic information about fetal age and tissue procurement procedures, including the form of abortion used, they impede further research.

Researchers may not deliberately withhold important details: they may not know, or may choose not to know, much about their source of fetal tissue. Nevertheless, the inconsistencies in the research findings may be related to the different sources of fetal tissue. One researcher may use tissue from a twelve-week-old fetus; another from a twenty-week-old fetus. Tissue may come from a miscarriage or a planned abortion or from an abortion done by vacuum aspiration or saline instillation. Until these and other details are routinely included in published articles, their importance cannot be assessed. Ironically, the publication of these details exposes scientists to the conflicts that have surrounded abortion clinics, and scientists, as well as physicians, do not want to become targets of militant Right-to-Life activists.

The procurement and transfer of fetal tissue costs money: a single transplant may require tissue from several, perhaps dozens, of fetuses. Individual fetuses often have too few nerve or liver cells to provide enough for the operation, and these cells must be carefully isolated from other cells, a task often made difficult by the process of abortion, which usually dismembers the fetus. Once collected these cells must be tested for genetic and other problems and stored until needed for research.

The idea of making a profit from collecting and selling fetal tissue, or any human tissue, is, to most people, repugnant. The Uniform Anatomical Gifts Act, a federal law, prohibits the sale of all human organs and tissues, including fetal tissue. Organ and tissue donation is supposed to be a gift, not a transaction—a rich patient is not allowed to outbid a poor one for an available kidney. But even those offended by the possibility of a tissue market might nonetheless agree that hospitals and clinics could reasonably be reimbursed for their expenses. The line between making profit and repaying costs is often hard to draw, however.

This issue has at least two dimensions: what expenses can be paid and who is eligible for reimbursement? Within limits— limits that have not yet been firmly set by regulation—tissue providers, most often abortion clinics, are allowed to include some of the costs of equipment and administrative overhead in the tissue costs. For many clinics, supplying fetal cells and tissue is an important source of income, even though in the narrow sense they do not profit from it. Women, who provide the tissue, are generally prohibited from being reimbursed for abortion expenses, however. In a continuing effort to keep the abortion decision separate from the use of the tissue after the abortion, clinics generally oppose any form of reimbursement for the mother. Such payment could become an incentive for abortion.

Even without financial incentives, however, the fear that procuring fetal tissue for research and treatment may influence abortion decisions haunts antiabortionists. The positive use of aborted remains may, to some, redeem the decision to end the pregnancy; if good can come from abortion, then abortion itself may, antiabortionists fear, be seen as a positive act.

It is also possible that someone would deliberately become pregnant not with the idea of having a child but to provide tissue needed to heal a loved one, or—and this is the worse nightmare of abortion foes—to sell the tissue. Sometime in the not too distant future, fetal tissue transplants may become a cure for a disease like Parkinson's. For a woman whose parent or husband suffers from this degenerative disease, becoming pregnant to provide fetal tissue for transplantation may, like offering a kidney, be a compelling moral obligation.

Moreover, if tissue is the woman's legal property and if not-for-profit organizations are paid for fetal tissue, what prohibits a woman from directly benefiting as well? Although many argue that few, if any, women would get pregnant merely to sell fetal tissue, a tissue market from poor nations around the world, especially those without ethical qualms about abortion, is a very real possibility. There have been at least two reports of women wanting to get pregnant to produce fetal tissue for transplant experiments: one wanted to help her parent with Alzheimer's disease and the other wanted to treat her own diabetes.[27] South Korea already supplies fetal tissue to researchers in other countries.

Most of the concerns about gathering and supplying of human fetal tissue remain hypothetical. Abuses, even isolated cases, have not been documented. Because of legal abortion, fetal tissue is plentiful. And since fetal tissue is much less immune-specific than adult tissue, matching donors and recipients will likely pose few problems, limiting pressure on individuals to donate tissue. No one is getting rich from fetal tissue, and American women are not becoming pregnant to sell their fetuses. Most suppliers and researchers responsibly collect and transfer the small amounts of fetal tissue needed for research.

But the demand for fetal tissue is currently low because the uses of fetal tissue are still experimental. If in the future fetal tissue transplantation becomes the treatment of choice of a common disease like diabetes, or even a rarer one like Parkinson's, then demand may outstrip supply. Fetal tissue may become a valuable and, perhaps, a scarce commodity, generating problems of procurement and supply.

4 The Search for Critical Definitions

Death, Life, Personhood

Antiabortion protesters often shout "Abortion is murder." The slogan makes a medical claim about the status of the fetus, a moral claim of fetal personhood, and a legal claim about fetal rights—all claims based on the belief that the fetus, regardless of level of development, is a person with the full complement of human rights.[1] But the definition of the fetus is ambiguous, and different groups hold very different views about its status.

Basing their views on the biology of development, scientists and physicians see the fetus in terms of its physical characteristics. Antiabortion activists start from a moral premise—a fetus is a person at conception—and argue that legal, medical, and scientific practice must build upon this foundation. The law, in mediating disputes, is concerned about the legal standing of the fetus; the point at which it becomes a person with full human rights. The relationship of fetal research to these questions of life, death, and personhood became the basis of the widely publicized trial, in 1973, of Dr. Kenneth Edelin.

*   *   *

On October 3, 1973, Dr. Kenneth Edelin performed a textbook abortion by hysterotomy at Boston City Hospital. Edelin performed the hysterotomy, a procedure similar to a cesarean section, after several previous attempts to induce the abortion by saline injection had failed. The mother had agreed to postpone her abortion for one day after consenting to participate in a fetal blood study. Edelin was not part of the research team studying fetal blood; he was the attending physician in charge of the abortion. During the abortion, Edelin surgically removed the fetus and sent the intact remains to the pathology department. (Unlike other forms of abortion, hysterotomies do not dismember the fetus.) To Dr. Edelin and his colleagues this was the end of a routine operation. There was nothing unusual about the case, no ethical dilemmas; it was just standard medical practice.

The case became everything but routine when, on April 1, 1974, the Grand Jury of Suffolk County, Boston, indicted Dr. Edelin of manslaughter. The operation occurred, ironically, nine months after the Supreme Court declared such abortions legal in its *Roe* v. *Wade* decision. But the Edelin trial was not over the legality of abortion, rather, it was over whether or when a fetus is a person who can be killed. The charge against Dr. Edelin was that he "did assault and beat a certain person, to wit: a male child described to the said JURORS as Baby Boy _____, and by such assault and beating did kill the said person."[2]

However, although the trial was not about abortion, this was clearly the issue. Having just lost in the Supreme Court, anti-abortion activists were looking for other battlefields where they could fight for their cause. The case against Dr. Edelin began when investigators confiscated the fetal remains of "Baby Boy _____" from the pathology department of Boston City Hospital while looking for evidence in the previously discussed grave-robbing case against the four doctors involved in the fetal metabolism study. The allegation of a medical resident, who was present during the hysterotomy and opposed to abortion, led to the manslaughter charge. He insisted that the fetus was alive after it was separated from the placenta and that Dr. Edelin had suffocated it before removing it from the mother.

The trial produced more confusion than clarity. Basic facts, such as the precise gestational age of the fetus or whether the fetus showed life signs—a beating heart or respiration—after it was separated from the placenta were disputed. Witnesses even disagreed on what it means to be born. Was the fetus born once it was detached from the placenta but still inside the womb? Or, does "born" mean disconnected from and outside the mother's body? Medically, the distinction involves only a matter of a few moments during an operation when the umbilical cord is cut and the fetus lifted from the womb. Legally, it can define the fetus as a living person.

This distinction was critical to the trial. After *Roe* v. *Wade,* the prosecution could not argue that the abortion was illegal; its case rested on the claim that this fetus was momentarily alive after the abortion procedure. Dr. Edelin was charged with manslaughter because he did not attempt to save the life of this allegedly born baby. As Judge James McGuire made clear to the jury, manslaughter occurs when someone unintentionally kills another and "the conduct of a defendant is so wanton or reckless in his act or the omission to act that it causes a death." Edelin knew that nothing could sustain the life signs of this nonviable fetus, and medical practice did not suggest reviving and sustaining its life signs. For the jury to find him guilty, it would have to define standard medical practice as "wanton and reckless" and the final stages of the hysterotomy as manslaughter.

In other words, a guilty verdict required defining a nonviable fetus aborted by hysterotomy as a born and living person who was then killed. The judge reviewed this point in great detail. He told the jurors,

> A fetus is not a person, and not the subject of an indictment
> for manslaughter. In order for a person to exist, he or she

must be born. Unborn persons, as I have said, are not the
subject of the crime of manslaughter. Birth is the process
which causes the emergence of a new individual from the
body of its mother. . . .

In order for the defendant to be found guilty in this case,
you must be satisfied beyond a reasonable doubt, as I have
defined that term for you, that the defendant caused the
death of a person who has been alive outside the body of
his or her mother.[3]

After hearing this charge and reviewing the evidence, the
unanimous jury found Dr. Edelin guilty. Even though the sentence was light (one year probation) and his conviction was
overturned in 1976, the manslaughter conviction of a doctor
who followed standard medical practice during a legal operation
sent shock waves through the medical and legal communities.
When confronted with the definitional questions of fetal viability, death, life, and personhood, a jury of twelve citizens
found that a twenty- to twenty-four-week-old fetus surgically
removed from its mother was a born person.

The Edelin jury based this decision less on the conflicting
expert testimony and medical arguments than on their image
of the fetus. During the trial the prosecutor showed, over the
objections of the defendant's lawyer, a picture of the fetus.
Science reporter Barbara Culliton described the response:

The jurors reported that they were shaken by the photo-
graph. "It looked like a baby," Liberty Ann Conlin told
reporters, ". . . it definitely had an effect on me." Paul Hol-
land commented, "The picture helped people draw their
own conclusions. Everyone in the room made up their minds
that the fetus was a person."[4]

The meaning of fetal life and death, and the biological, legal,
and ethical differences between the early fetus wholly dependent on the pregnant woman and the more developed fetus that
could survive outside the womb are, as the Edelin trial so pain-

fully illustrates, questions of bitter dispute. Different groups—scientists, physicians, antiabortionists, women's rights advocates, legal scholars, and judges—offer different answers, and the political furor that engulfed fetal research is fueled by their incommensurable views. Three central definitional problems compound the dispute over personhood: the meanings of fetal death, of life, and of viability.

Definitions of fetal death, life, and viability are elusive for a number of reasons. They cannot be defined or even discussed without addressing the status of pregnant women; questions about fetal personhood are inseparable from a woman's personhood.[5] Nor are they meaningful without reference to each other. In American society, we acknowledge anyone who is born as being alive but define death as the absence of certain physical characteristics. This confounds the state of the unborn fetus; for it is not clear at what point we can meaningfully say that it is alive as a person.

The biological ambiguity of the fetus has several dimensions. The fetus is both separate from, yet part of, the woman who carries it. It is unseen, except through technical means of the sonogram or embryoscope, yet present. Long before it is felt moving in the womb the presence of the fetus radically alters the woman's body. Unlike other cells or organs, the fetus has its own individual genetic heritage and the potential to become an individual. Nevertheless, a young fetus is dependent on the woman who carries it and in its early stages cannot live outside the womb despite all current and anticipated medical advances.

Inside the womb, the fetus changes rapidly, developing in a few months, if all goes well, from a few microscopic cells to a born baby. At what stage do those microscopic cells become a human being? Some argue that a fetus is fully human at the moment of conception and, therefore, stages of development should make no difference to how it is perceived and treated.[6] Sissela Bok counters that biological differences between an undeveloped fetus and an older, more developed fetus change the ethical issues: "[Early fetal cells] cannot feel the anguish or pain connected with death. . . . Words such as 'harm' or 'deprive' cannot be meaningfully used in the context of early abortion and fetal development."[7]

But where is the line between a developed and undeveloped fetus? The biological differences between an early embryo and a near-term fetus are immeasurable, greater than the differences between a newborn and an adult. But what of the difference between an eighteen- and a twenty-week-old fetus? It is difficult, perhaps meaningless, to infer fine distinctions from the vast changes made during fetal development. Development is a continuous process with few definite thresholds about which we can make clear-cut moral and medical distinctions.[8] Stages or steps along the developmental continuum are always arbitrary.[9]

These definitional ambiguities are one source of the fetal research controversy. To use the fetus for purposes of research requires distinctions between living and dead and viable and nonviable life. And such distinctions must be acceptable to groups with very different values.

Between life and death is a zone of ambiguity. There is little social dispute over standards of treatment for the obviously alive and the obviously dead; no one confuses surgery with autopsy. But the line dividing alive from dead is not biological. We do not define death as the complete end of biological activity, because many bodily functions—digestion, hair growth, cell division—continue long after someone is declared dead. When we say someone is dead we mean that the body no longer "holds" the person.

While depending on medical or biological evidence, definitions of death are infused with social meaning; death has profound policy implications, bearing on the division of estates, the use of organs, and, for our purposes, the nature of research. Declaring death assumes agreement on the features humans must have that distinguish living from dead persons, as well as on cultural and religious concepts of death and personhood.[10] These definitions change with the times, often as a result of scientific advances.

In 1968, a committee of the Harvard Medical School faculty, responding to medical advances, issued a report redefining death. They proposed the now standard brain-death criteria. Prior to 1968, the legal definition of death meant the cessation of pulse and respiration, as determined by a physician.[11] The popular image of the doctor rushing to the scene, feeling the pulse, and declaring death accurately portrayed the consensus.

Medical progress in reviving and then sustaining these life signs challenged this definition. Were patients whose bodies were kept alive by modern technology alive or dead? Is it murder if a patient dies after the machines are shut off? Is someone alive if the upper brain no longer functions but the brain stem keeps the heart beating? The promise of organ transplants added urgency to these ethical difficulties. If doctors needed to wait for the heart to stop, then kidneys or other organs might no longer be useful for transplantation.

The Harvard group defined brain death as the end of all functioning in both the upper and lower brain. In effect, they added a new clinical criteria to the heart-lung standard, since a brain-dead patient cannot sustain pulse and breath if disconnected from life-support. By measuring brain waves, doctors could declare someone dead even while mechanically maintaining traditional life signs. Brain death has become the standard medical and legal definition of death.

Although this redefinition of death shifted attention from the heart to the brain, central aspects of the definition of death remained the same. First is the issue of authority: doctors define death. The change in medical criteria did not require a change in law since the law treats death as a fact defined by physicians.[12]

Second, the brain-death criteria does not equate death with the end of cognition: it relies on a whole brain criteria. If the patient has lost all cerebral functioning but the brain stem keeps the heart beating and the lungs breathing, the person is considered alive. Karen Anne Quinlan lived for several years in this way after she was removed from life-support systems, but she never regained consciousness. Others have argued for the narrower standards of cerebral or neocortical death.[13] These standards equate higher brain functioning—awareness, feeling, thinking—with minimal human characteristics and would allow physicians to declare someone in an irreversible vegetative state, such as Karen Anne Quinlan, dead.

This less conservative view has implications for the treatment of anencephalic newborns, stroke victims, and advanced cases of Alzheimer's disease. But for now, death of a child or adult means the complete cessation of brain activity, and this definition has important implications for considering fetal life and death and for the availability of the fetus for research.

Defining fetal death proves more difficult than defining the death of a child or an adult. First, it is not clear when a fetus can be considered alive as a person, a topic discussed momentarily. Without consensus on the beginning of life, how do you define its end? Second, there are significant biological differences between an early- and late-term fetus and between a fetus and a neonate which raise doubt about applying standards to a fetus that are reasonable for a child.

Young fetuses have not yet developed circulatory, respiratory, or nervous systems, and this greatly complicates the task of applying medical standards of death, whether heart-lung or brain-death standards. A beating heart is present in a one-month-old embryo, but the heart pumps no blood since the circulation system has not yet developed. This early heart is merely a rhythmically contracting cluster of cells. By the beginning of the fourth month, a fetus can move its chest enough to pull amniotic fluid in and out of the respiratory tract, but most fetuses born even at six months cannot sustain respiration.

A twenty-two-week fetal brain is smooth, lacking the complex folds that become evident from thirty-six weeks on. A ten-week-old fetus squints, opens and closes its mouth, and flexes its fingers and toes. Sucking begins at six months. The integration of the nervous and muscular functions proceeds rapidly from the beginning of the third trimester. Some neurological developments, such as color and shape perception, do not occur until long after birth.

Basic differences in fetal cells and tissues may also change the meaning of death. For a child or an adult brief interruptions in breathing and heartbeat quickly lead to irreparable nerve damage. Without abundant oxygen, brain and nerve cells atrophy, causing permanent damage. In a fetus, brain death may be less permanent. A fetus is much more resistant to oxygen deprivation and, except late in term, nerve cells can grow to replace damaged ones. Indeed, this very property encourages researchers to see promise in fetal nerve tissue grafts as a cure for degenerative brain diseases.

Fetuses, even late-term fetuses, are, however, more susceptible to hypothermia than neonates. Premature infants maintain core body temperature with great difficulty, while fetuses younger than twenty-two weeks are almost "cold-blooded," relying on their womb environment to maintain their temperature.[14] Signs of fetal death are masked by hypothermia and may be reversed when the fetus is returned to normal body temperature.[15] Thus, it is possible that a young fetus could sustain some life signs for extended periods if kept warm. But is such a fetus dead or alive?

An aspect of fetal death that is central to the controversy over fetal research is that most fetuses that are used in research did not die accidentally. For reasons discussed later, research cannot depend on miscarriages, stillbirths, and ectopic pregnancies; fetal research largely depends on induced abortions. One does not need to take sides in the abortion dispute to acknowledge that planned abortion involves a decision to end a pregnancy that might end in a live birth. Abortion is intentional, and many argue that the intentional foreclosure of the possibility for life changes the ethical context of fetal research.

Moreover, the process of abortion most commonly obliterates any signs of life. Aborted fetuses are usually torn apart during evacuation, leaving no discernible body to test for respiration, circulation, or brain waves; nurses often need to inventory the disembodied fetal body parts to be sure that the abortion was complete.[16] Occasionally fetuses aborted by hysterotomy result in intact, nearly viable fetuses that demonstrate fleeting heartbeat and nervous system activity, but most abortions eliminate all life signs. Thus, for many fetuses, the abortion itself is the criterion for death.[17]

A developing fetus is biologically alive. It grows and changes rapidly, but these characteristics do not make it alive as a person. Prior to conception sperm and egg cells are just as surely biologically alive; even life-threatening cancer cells grow and change. Moreover, any cell or tissue, healthy or cancerous, is distinctly human: it does not belong to another species. Just as declaring death depends on the absence of features that we consider essential to personhood, declaring the moment life begins requires identifying when the characteristics of personhood are first present. The views are often polarized: life begins at birth or life begins at conception. But there is also an intermediate view, the brain-alive theory.

The view that life begins at birth solves many definitional problems. Birth is a recognizable stage that clearly marks a significant step in life. To define the beginning of life at birth accepts that a fetus is biologically alive and that, especially later in pregnancy, it shares many characteristics with a baby. However, while recognizing the fetus as a potential or developing human being, it reserves full human status until the moment of separation from the mother.

This view has a long cultural heritage. We measure life span in birthdays. For centuries, English law has identified birth as the moment human life begins.[18] In the U.S., doctors record births when the infant is separated from the mother and shows life signs such as breathing, heartbeat, or voluntary muscle movements. Stillbirths and abortions do not require birth or death certificates, and the "birth" of a previable fetus is labeled a miscarriage. Many feminists support the view that life begins at birth, stressing the complete dependence of the fetus on the woman.

The Connecticut Supreme Court recently reinforced this view.[19] The justices unanimously ruled that a pregnant woman who injected cocaine just before giving birth was not guilty of child abuse and ordered that the state return her child; a healthy three-year-old who was taken from the mother at birth. To the justices, the drug-using mother was not guilty of child abuse because prior to birth the fetus was not yet a child.

At the same time, changes in tort law and prebirth child neglect cases are eroding the consensus that life, or at least legal life, begins at birth. Although the moment of birth signals important physical changes, most notably the independence of the circulation system, the differences between a near-term fetus and a neonate are slight. In a period when cesarean deliveries are common, birth dates are often determined by the physician's and parents' appointment books rather than by any developmental changes in the fetus. Moreover, the near-term fetus clearly shows heart and brain activity: if not alive, it is surely not dead.

The view that life begins at conception takes another biological milestone—the sperm fertilizing the egg—as the beginning of human life. Again we are faced with the same problem. Clearly a fertilized egg is living and human, but so is an unfertilized egg. Fertilization marks the creation of a new genetic identity, but are we willing to say that a zygote is a person? Antiabortion activists unequivocally answer "yes." Indeed, throughout the 1970s and early 1980s, antiabortion members of Congress promoted a pro-life amendment to the Constitution that declared in the first sentence: "The Congress finds that the life of each human being begins at Conception."[20] This amendment never passed but would have reversed *Roe* v. *Wade* by declaring a newly formed embryo a citizen with Fourteenth Amendment rights.

Some advocates of the view that life begins at conception argue that all the ingredients of a person are present at conception and that genes determine human nature. The mother provides only nutriment and protection to the fetus, permitting, in effect, the already determined person to realize his or her self. This view equates personhood with a unique set of genes, since at conception the fertilized egg is little more than forty-six newly scrambled chromosomes containing the genetic codes that guide development.

Most scientists reject this rigid, deterministic view of development and instead describe the genetic code as containing many potentials.[21] They describe development as emergent, not predetermined; the individual fetus arises out of a complex interaction of genes, maternal influence, and chance. It is also not clear when this process begins or ends. The development of a genetically unique individual begins long before fertilization with the creation of the egg and sperm cells through the cell-division process of meiosis, and this process began when our genetic parents were themselves fetuses.[22] While still in the womb, our biological mothers developed approximately six million egg cells by their sixth fetal month. This number is cut drastically to two million by birth, after which no further eggs are produced. The male fetus develops germ cells called spermatogonia, which increase in number until birth but remain dormant until puberty when they begin sperm production.

It is also not clear exactly when conception occurs. The sperm and egg do not exchange chromosomes until approximately twenty-four hours after the sperm has entered the egg. After the genetic material is combined, the embryo (or what some biologists call the "pre-embryo") begins the process of division and differentiation. At the earliest stages when the embryo consists of four to eight cells, each cell has the potential to form an entire individual—they are totipotential—but as soon as differentiation begins the cells lose this capacity. It is not biologically clear, therefore, if the embryo is genetically unique before or after differentiation. Genetic identity is not, however, a sufficient definition of a person, since identical twins are considered two persons even though they are genetic duplicates, and the placenta is not granted person status even though it shares the genetic code of the fetus it helped nourish.[23]

In addition, the creation of a genetically distinct individual does not assure development. The natural mortality of embryos is very high; approximately 85 percent die at some point in the journey toward birth, most before implantation in the uterine wall.[24] Conception is a milestone, but genetics offer no clear answer to the question of when human life begins. One cannot take a zygote, raise it in an artificial womb, and expect a baby to crawl out of the lab.

In addition to overstating the significance of fertilization and understating the interaction of the fetus and its environment in the womb, the view that life begins at conception creates innumerable legal conundrums. Common contraceptives, such as the IUD and the pill, work, in part, by preventing implantation, not conception.[25] Such devices would be murder weapons if life began at conception, because they kill the embryo by preventing it from attaching to the lining of the uterus. Indeed, this was one basis for opposition to the RU-486 morning-after pill.

Procedures for in vitro fertilization could also lead to charges of mass murder. Typically a number of eggs are fertilized and then allowed to develop in the lab before the healthiest is surgically implanted in the mother. The remaining embryos are either returned to cold storage for future implantation or are thrown away; neither alternative would be appropriate treatment for a person with Fourteenth Amendment protected rights. A recent court case, brought by a father who refused to allow his divorced wife to have custody of lab-fertilized eggs, underscored the social and legal confusion that will result from defining conception as life.[26] Should this divorced couple be forced to raise all of these embryos? Who has the legal right to keep them?

Defining the beginning of human life or personhood at either birth or conception benefits from simplicity, being based on specific and easily recognized events. But both views ignore the complexity and significance of fetal development. To find a milestone, a point, during the stages of fetal development when the fetus becomes an alive person may not be possible.[27]

Nevertheless, there are efforts to use brain activity as a standard for beginning of life. This approach offers an appealing symmetry: if we now define death as the absence of whole brain functioning, then we could define life as the emergence of whole brain activity. Like brain death, defining brain life suggests there are medically determined criteria. And to the scientific community this has the added benefit of removing the definition from political and legal conflict.[28]

The beginning of brain life cannot, however, be established by merely reversing brain death. Brain death is measured by a flat electroencephalogram (EEG), but in a fetus neural functioning emerges gradually. Nerve activity begins early, with the nervous system beginning to function at about eight weeks. At this early stage of development the fetus turns its head when touched around the mouth. However, this level of brain development does not signify the fetus is alive. Brain death means that the brain can no longer sustain circulation and breathing, but even though the nervous system has begun to function, an eight-week-old fetus has not yet developed these activities.

By eighteen to twenty weeks, the nervous system is substantially developed. Clifford Grobstein summarizes neural development at this age as "roughly comparable to . . . the stable comatose state displayed by Karen Anne Quinlan, a state just short of the current definition of brain death."[29] But, unlike Karen Anne Quinlan, who lived for years once removed from life-support systems, a twenty-week-old fetus could not survive once separated from the life-support of the womb. Independent survivability waits for further development of the respiration and metabolic systems. Even if the brain is ready, the rest of the fetus is not.

Brain-dead adults and brain-not-yet-alive fetuses also differ in another significant way. Brain-dead adults lack consciousness and cannot feel pain; they cannot physically suffer. It is not clear at what point a fetus feels pain. It is reasonable to assume that sensation and subjective awareness do not exist before some level of neural maturation, when synaptic connectivity and neurotransmitter activity reach a threshold.[30] Although it is not clear when a fetus develops sensation, rudimentary sensation occurs long before the stage when the nervous system can keep a fetus alive.

It is probable that advances in science will better pinpoint the stages when a fetus develops sensation, feeling, and even awareness. At this point, all that can be said with confidence is that there are no specific development milestones that establish the moment when a fetus becomes brain-alive. Our last definitional problem, however, does have a clear biological base.

Fetal viability is a critical concept, defining the medical and legal threshold for research on the fetus. The working definition of fetal viability depends on the level of fetal development and current medical practice. A viable fetus can live outside the womb; it can sustain independent life. A nonviable fetus is not yet sufficiently developed to biologically survive despite the best efforts of physicians.[31]

Viability is more than a biological concept, however. A full-term newborn requires extraordinary efforts from adults to feed and protect it; its early life is only slightly less dependent than it was in the womb. The term "independent" is, therefore, misleading. Moreover, a definition of viability must address the question of "how long" the fetus must survive outside the womb before it is considered viable: need it survive a few minutes or several days?

According to the current medical definition of viability, the fetus must be sufficiently advanced to survive and develop outside the womb into an infant even though this survival may require extraordinary medical intervention, including life-support. For a fetus at the threshold of viability, survivability is rare, not guaranteed or even likely. A non- or not-yet-viable fetus is medically similar to a dying adult whose life signs cannot be sustained even with the most advanced life-support systems. Not-yet-viable fetuses lack the organ systems, especially the lungs and neurological integration, to sustain life. Although the precise definitions vary, fetuses younger than twenty-two weeks and weighing less than 500 grams are considered *non*viable.

The definition of viability is medically conservative; the probability that a fetus that weighs between 600 and 700 grams or between 1.3 and 1.5 pounds will survive is slim. According to medical records, the smallest infant who survived weighed about 400 grams, or less than one pound.[32] This medical anomaly was recorded in 1939, and the infant was weighed on a grocery scale, leading most doctors to doubt the accuracy of the report. In a study of 160,000 deliveries that occurred between 1956 and 1980, the smallest infant to survive weighed 580 grams. Out of the 121,000 deliveries in another study, only two infants weighing less than 700 grams survived. Of these, the smaller weighed 540 grams and the infant was probably more developed than the low weight suggested. Another study examined 250 babies born in Providence, Rhode Island, between 1977 and 1981 and weighing between 500 and 1,000 grams. None of those weighing less than 600 grams survived, and only three percent weighing between 600 and 700 grams survived.[33]

The current viability standard is, therefore, set not at the point where fetal long-term survivability is rare, but at the point where it is considered medically impossible. Most scientific standards are based on probability: the risk of accidents or hazards is considered remote but greater than zero. Fetal viability is, from a medical point of view, an absolute standard; a nonviable fetus has no chance of survival at all. Extremely premature infants, those near the viability threshold, have little chance of survival, and those that do survive often suffer mental retardation and other birth defects. Nonetheless, physicians try to save the lives of viable fetuses.

One reason viability is defined so conservatively is that fetal age cannot be precisely determined. While still in the womb, the best measure of age is the length from the top of the head to the base of the spine, the crown-rump length. This measure requires a sonogram and must take into account the relatively wide normal variation of fetal sizes. Once outside the womb weight can be measured precisely, but poorly nourished, unhealthy fetuses or unusually small fetuses are often more developed than their size suggests.

Medical care for premature infants has greatly improved over the last twenty-five years: neonatal mortality in the U.S. decreased from 20.5 per 1,000 live births in 1950 to 9.4 in 1978.[34] The age of viability, however, has changed only slightly during the twentieth century. Although he did not use the term "viable," in 1903 J. Whitridge Williams describes, in the first edition of *Obstetrics,* the ages when a fetus is likely to survive. At six months or twenty-four weeks, Williams wrote, "A foetus born at this period will attempt to breathe and move its limbs, but always perishes within a short time."[35] At the end of the seventh month, the first edition notes a slight chance of survival: "A foetus born at this period moves it limbs quite energetically and cries with a weak voice; but, as a rule, it cannot be raised, even with the most expert care, although an occasional successful case is found in the records."[36]

The language in the eighteenth edition of the same text— editions that span eighty-seven years of remarkable medical progress in the care of pregnant women and newborns—echoes the first. The 1989 edition states that at six months, "A fetus born at this period will attempt to breathe but almost always dies shortly after birth."[37] The qualifier "almost" is the only substantive change. The 1989 edition is, however, more optimistic at seven months than its 1903 predecessor: "An infant born at this time in gestation moves his or her limbs quite energetically and cries weakly. The infant of this gestational age, with expert care, most often will survive."[38]

Medical researchers have tried to develop new life support systems for fetuses younger than twenty weeks. Some have predicted a time when fertilized eggs can be incubated outside the womb and fetuses can be nurtured in an artificial placenta, but most medical researchers and physicians doubt that the age of fetal viability will be greatly reduced.[39] Experiments immersing fetuses between twenty- and twenty-four-weeks gestational age in hyper-oxygenated fluid were able to briefly sustain life signs: some for nearly twenty-four hours. These experiments done in the early 1970s helped spark the fetal research controversy, since keeping nonviable fetuses alive to test equipment struck many as unconscionable. The very limited success of these and similar experiments indicates that the medical definition of fetal viability is unlikely to change for the foreseeable future.

Although fetal viability is a medical concept—doctors define when a fetus can survive outside the womb—it is also a legal milestone. Nowhere is this more evident than in the *Roe* v. *Wade* abortion ruling. When considering the conflict between a woman's right to privacy and self-determination and the fetus's right to state protection, the Supreme Court made the three-tiered decision based on viability; prior to fetal viability near the end of the second trimester the fetus has no legal standing. The Court rejected the antiabortion claim that "abortion is murder" by declaring that a previable fetus is not a legal person and could not, therefore, be killed.

Ultimately any definition of life is only partially biological, and developmental changes are inevitably interpreted according to metaphysical and moral beliefs. The beginning or end of fetal life cannot be defined with certainty or consensus. The sustained confusion is both biological and cultural; there are no unambiguous developmental milestones that separate fetal life from nonlife, nor is there a social consensus on the features that signify the threshold of life. We are left with fetal viability as the medical and legal working definition of the beginning of human life, although opponents of fetal research reject as immoral the belief that a previable fetus is not a person.

This unresolvable definitional problem is the root cause of the fetal research dispute. With no agreement on the meaning of fetal life and death, public policy concerning the funding of fetal experiments and the regulation of fetal tissue transplants is built on a foundation of shifting sand. No one can build a breakwater to shore up these definitions; ambiguity is fundamental.

5 Fetus as Tissue, Fetus as Person

For the jurors in the Edelin trial the image of the fetus as a baby defined the issue and guided their decision to charge the doctor with manslaughter; this trial and the subsequent controversy over fetal research have been shaped by conflicting images of the fetus.

In a minimalist view, the nonviable fetus is little more than a form of the pregnant woman's bodily tissue: it is part of the woman without separate identity or status. This image of the fetus as tissue de-emphasizes the importance of the fetus's separate genetic identity and is most tenable in the early gestational stages.

This is the view of the nonviable fetus that dominates medical practice. Fetal remains are most commonly discarded in the same manner as other by-products of surgery.[1] Fetal remains do not receive death certificates—they are not dead in the eyes of the state—nor are they buried or cremated. With no moral status, they are simply thrown away.

For the small percentage of fetal remains that are used in research, the definition of the fetus as tissue also dominates procurement and distribution procedures. Most researchers who rely on fetal tissue or cells develop direct relations with hospitals and abortion clinics. Rarely are pregnant women asked to give specific consent on the use of fetal tissue. Women choosing abortion customarily sign a blanket consent form that is similar, if not identical, to general surgery consents. These forms often contain one phrase among the many disclaimers such as "I further understand that in accordance with applicable law, any tissue removed may be disposed of in accordance with the custom practiced."[2]

In some cases, consent forms may inform the woman that the fetus may be examined and used in research, but specific consent is the exception, not the norm.[3] In the late 1980s, the president of a nonprofit supplier of fetal tissue asked clinics and hospitals to require informed consent from the mother for the use of tissue in research. Approximately half of these medical centers stopped supplying him fetal tissue: informed consent was too much trouble.[4] Consent for the use of fetal tissue is often considered unnecessary hospital red tape.

Routine medical practice, then, codifies the image of the nonviable fetus as tissue, raising a moral point that Representative Henry Waxman captured in an ironic comment about the opposition to fetal research:

> Whatever else is done with the tissue from legal abortions, no one should learn anything from it. Don't research it, don't study it, don't find cures for disease from it. Instead, unlike a lifesaving organ transplant from a brain-dead adult, the fetal tissue will just be buried.[5]

If the aborted fetus is the tissue by-product of legal surgery, it would, in this view, be wrong to merely discard it when it could be used to advance medical science and perhaps medical treatment. The image of the fetus as tissue not only justifies its use in research and medicine but makes the moral claim that discarding fetal tissue is an immoral waste, that not to use it is wrong.

A variation on this image of fetus as tissue is the view that the fetus is property. The nature of tissue property rights varies depending on how the fetus is defined. If the dead fetus is considered a dead person, then legal tradition and precedent gives family members only "quasi-property rights": the right to dispose of the body but not the right to sell or profit from it.[6]

If, on the other hand, the fetus is a pregnant woman's tissue, then the full range of property rights might apply. Reviewing the law and legal precedent, Nancy Field concludes:

> A uniform and absolute legal distinction between fetal and other bodily tissue does not presently exist. . . . [F]rom a legal perspective, once a pre-viable fetus is dead, it possesses no rights and is not recognized by the courts as a juridical entity.[7]

Legal tradition concurs with current medical practice that a dead, previable fetus is maternal tissue. Extending full property rights to the mother over her fetal tissue is a logical, but for some a disturbing extension of this view. Full property rights include not only the right to dispose of the body but also the right to profit directly from the sale of tissue and indirectly from royalties earned from drugs and treatments derived from the tissue.

A recent court case in California, *Moore* v. *The Regents of the University of California,* generated a debate about according full tissue property rights to women.[8] John Moore was a leukemia patient at UCLA, where part of his spleen was removed. His spleen, doctors discovered, could produce a substance that builds resistance to leukemia. The cell line from Moore's spleen was patented and sold to several pharmaceutical firms. Moore had never given consent to this use of his spleen and, when contacted, refused to wave his property interests. Instead, he sued. Following the standard view in the law of granting people only "quasi-property rights" over tissue, the original court did not grant standing, but in July 1988, the appeals court did agree that Moore had a property interest in his tissue. The court eventually ruled against Moore, but the claim itself suggested that researchers and drug companies might share their profits with tissue donors. For antiabortionists, this raised the specter that financial incentives would encourage abortion, the "harvesting of babies" for sale.

These images of the fetus, or at least the previable fetus, as tissue or property both stress the dependence of the fetus on the pregnant woman. But the fetus is not a spleen. Though wholly dependent on the pregnant woman and unable to live outside her womb, a not-yet-viable fetus is genetically distinct from the pregnant woman; it is not an organ or tissue, but a body, suggesting to some that it can be defined as a person.

The images of the fetus as a person or baby de-emphasize its dependence on the pregnant woman and its lack of physical development, stressing instead its overall form. These images have long traditions in Western culture: medieval anatomists, copying from Roman drawings, portrayed the fetus as a miniature adult encased in the womb (see Figure 5-1).[9] These early scientists knew that newborns and fetuses do not look like adults; their unrealistic portraits illustrated their culturally defined image of the fetus as a person, not an anatomically accurate representation which eventually became more common during the Renaissance.

Later portraits of the fetus, from Leonardo da Vinci's drawings to intrauterine photographs, also convey the image of the fetus as a baby. After eleven gestational weeks, the fetus has the shape of a baby: the large head with some facial features, the arms and legs, the discernible hand (see Figure 5-2). The view that the fetus is tissue or tissue property is founded on complex scientific evidence about human development and legal arguments about torts and rights, whereas the image of the fetus as a baby is based on a simple, emotional reaction to the form: it looks like a baby.[10]

Sonograms reinforce this image of the fetus as a grown baby.

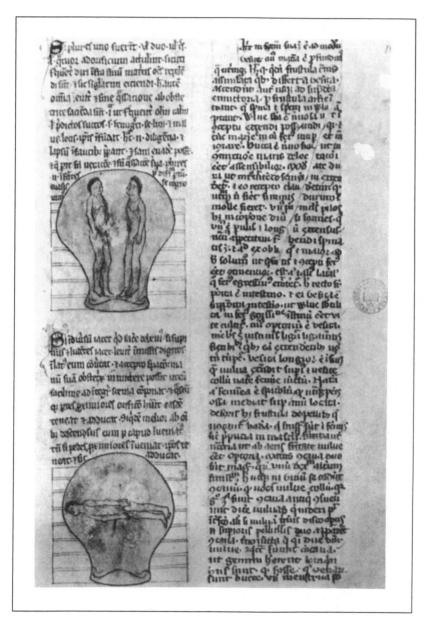

FIG. 5-1. *Fetus as Miniature Adult as Depicted in Thirteenth-Century English Manuscript*

Reprinted by permission from T. V. N. Persaud, *Early History of Human Anatomy: From Antiquity to the Beginning of the Modern Era* (Springfield, IL: Charles C. Thomas, 1984), 83. From the collection of the Clendening History of Medicine Library, The University of Kansas Medical Center.

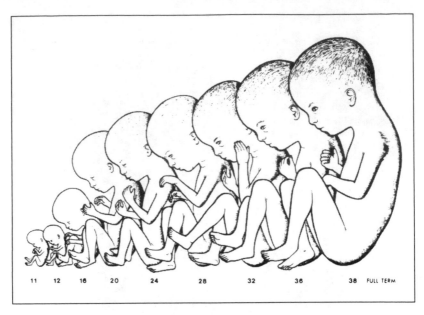

FIG. 5-2. *Modern Views of the Development of the Fetus*

Reprinted by permission from Jack A. Pritchard and Paul C. MacDonald, *Williams Obstetrics,* 16th edition (New York: Appleton-Century-Crofts, 1980), 173.

Although not a medical necessity in most pregnancies, sonograms have become routine, giving parents a glimpse of the moving, pulsating fetus long before it is felt in the womb. Sonograms turn the abstraction of pregnancy into a real image of the fetus. Prior to the sonogram the early fetus was imagined, or it was felt but not seen. The sonogram provides a visual image; it is not uncommon for parents to paste a sonogram snapshot in their baby album, or to make the image into Christmas cards.

One mother retells her fascination while seeing a sonogram of her fetus.

> At first, it is hard to make sense of the swirling, unstable pattern of light and dark, but when the fetus is still, one can soon distinguish its head and then, a little less clearly, its torso. . . . I, at least, was unprepared to see that figure emerge from the initially unintelligible swirls, unprepared for the knowledge that I was looking at my baby specifically as it was at that very moment. The picture shocked me, as though I had broken a taboo, thrilled me for the extension of my powers, surprised me by its concrete actuality. . . .[11]

The image of the fetus as a baby provides those opposed to abortion and fetal research with a powerful symbol, supporting their belief that personhood begins at conception. When Dr. Edelin was tried for manslaughter of a fetus, prosecutors fought to have pictures of fetuses introduced as evidence. Antiabortion protesters carry posters of babylike fetuses, and fetal research opponents denounce the images of fetuses immersed in fish tanks and severed fetal heads.

Nowhere is this visual rhetoric more powerful than in the Right-to-Life film *The Silent Scream.* Based largely on sonogram images, this movie purports to show a fetus panic and then scream before an impending abortion. According to its critics, the film is skillful propaganda, edited to coordinate random fetal movements with the abortion. Young fetuses cannot anticipate, scream, or even feel pain, so the medical experts argue. But scientific rebuttals do not blunt the symbolic impact of the images conveyed by the film of the fetus as a frightened baby anticipating its own death.[12]

Although not to the extent advocated by antiabortion activists, the *Roe* decision actually granted the late-term fetus greater legal status than it traditionally received. In this the Court was acknowledging recent legal trends. In the past, legal rights began at birth. The Fourteenth Amendment of the Constitution begins "All persons born or naturalized in the United States . . . are citizens of the United States. . . ." Prior to 1946, tort cases required that the baby be born before assessing liability and damages; therefore, in the past you could not be held liable for injury to the fetus.

This tradition is changing. Seventeen states now define the crime of murder of an unborn child, but the murder can occur only after viability.[13] Indiana and Arizona are the only states that impose criminal liability for the wrongful death of a fetus at any stage of development.[14] Third parties are increasingly held liable for damage to the fetus; for example, in many jurisdictions if a woman pregnant with a viable fetus dies in an auto accident, the person responsible is charged with two counts of manslaughter. A Michigan court even allowed a child to sue his mother for the discoloration of his teeth caused by her taking tetracycline during pregnancy.[15]

The courts are also extending child protection and child abuse and neglect statutes to late-term pregnancies. One case involved a twenty-nine-year-old pregnant woman who was sent to jail for forging $700 in checks: rather than give her the usual probation, the court incarcerated her to protect her fetus from her cocaine habit.[16]

Since 1981, there have been at least twenty-one requests for court-ordered cesarean sections.[17] In these cases, as with a smaller number of court-ordered fetal surgeries, the fetus is treated in court like an abused or neglected child. The fetus and the mother are opponents in court each represented by an attorney; the fetus is assigned an attorney *ad litem*. If the court decides for the fetus, as it did in eighteen of the twenty-one cesarean section cases, the state takes temporary custody of the fetus while it is still in the womb and requires that the woman submit to the operation.[18] In a recent case in Chicago, however, the court refused to force Mircea Bricci to have a cesarean, which was against her religious beliefs; the hospital insisted that the fetus was not getting enough oxygen and would likely die without the operation. Her baby, Callian, weighed less than five pounds at birth but otherwise seemed healthy.[19]

A New York court recently added a new twist. In *Gloria C. v. William C.* the court awarded the pregnant Gloria C., her two children, and her fetus separate protective orders from her abusive husband, William C. Acting as if the abusive husband could threaten the fetus without going near the mother, the court held "that a fetus is a person for the purpose of issuing a protective order."[20]

In contrast to these cesarean section cases, most fetuses used in research are not living, but those who see the fetus as a person consider the dead fetus as a corpse, not discarded tissue. A dead fetus is, in this view, best seen as a cadaver or cadaverous tissue donor. A corpse is not a living person and does not warrant the level of care granted the living. But as a total physical remnant of a person, it receives different treatment than tissue discarded during surgery.

Although they no longer have protected legal interests, the dead are traditionally treated with a respect not given to tissue fragments.[21] For example, corpses are not used in car crash tests without specific persmission of next of kin, not because these tests will harm the corpse but because they violate norms of respectful treatment; a corpse is not a crash dummy even though neither is alive. But most fetal remains are not intact bodies, and rarely in American society are fetal corpses given ceremonies common to dead children or adults.

Yet the use of dead fetuses as tissue and organ donors raises important symbolic and value questions associated with the respectful treatment of the dead. Procedures for tissue and organ donation from adult corpses honor the importance of autonomy and individualism to American society.[22] A person is granted control over his or her body after death so that in most states the donor needs to indicate a willingness to donate. But this value does not apply to the fetal corpse since it never achieved autonomy. Family interest is also important. Next of kin are traditionally given the right to dispose of the body, even, at times, overriding the expressed concern of the deceased. Although many antiabortion activists insist that the abortion decision nullifies all kinship rights, it is hard to argue that parents forfeit legal rights over the disposal of the body as long as abortion is legal.

Donation of tissue and organs is generally viewed as a gift. When a person donates blood or a sibling gives another a kidney, no money is asked for or given.[23] Clearly the corpse is not aware of the gift, but the value of giving rather than selling is central to the social acceptance of tissue and organ donations. Although money is often exchanged to cover costs and many not-for-profit arrangements are highly lucrative, buying and selling body parts, whether adult or fetal, is ethically repellent in part because organ donation implies a kind of transformation or redemption. Often the opportunity for organ donation follows tragedy, a fatal accident, for example. Family members, who authorize donating eyes, kidneys, or other organs, often describe these gifts as redeeming the tragedy, of making some good come out of a bad event. Although rarely seen as a direct motive for donation, the very act of donation transforms loss into a means to help another.

In the case of fetal organ donation, this value is especially troubling to abortion's opponents. They fear the redemptive power of donation. If donating fetal tissue for medical research or treatment relieves some of the anguish of the decision to have an abortion, this would weaken their moral stand against abortion. And, if the result of donating fetal tissue is viewed as positive, this could actually encourage abortion. Faced with a tragic family situation—a parent suffering from Alzheimer's or

Parkinson's, a child with a spinal cord injury, a pregnant sister with a history of transmitting a genetic disease—that could be treated with a fetal tissue transplant, the power to heal could encourage abortion when none was considered. Thus, anti-abortionists reject the image of the fetus as a cadaverous organ donor, and they strongly oppose the use of fetal tissue in trans-plantation research. Although considering the previable fetus as an organ or tissue donor gives it greater status than viewing it as mere tissue, the moral politics of the antiabortion move-ment rejects, ironically, this limited form of fetal "personhood."

Another form of "personhood" is "patienthood." The image of the fetus as a patient relies less on the visual image and more on developments in medical practice. Traditionally, the woman, not the fetus, was the primary patient in prenatal care, except, perhaps, in the very last stages of pregnancy. Obstetricians, and midwives before them, often spoke of having two patients, the mother and the unborn baby, but when there was a conflict between the mother's and the fetus's health, the mother's med-ical needs, with rare exception, took precedent.

This is still the case. Even strong antiabortion activists gen-erally consent to early abortions that would save the pregnant woman's life. However, medical advances, many based on fetal research, have brought us to the point where, "the fetus, once a captive of its own environment, an enigma to be protected but left untreated, finally has gained the status of patient."[24]

6 Fetus as Patient

Because of improved medical care for both the pregnant woman and the fetus and advances in fetal imaging, the fetus is being treated more often as an independent patient. Pregnancy was, until recently, life-threatening to many women, as a visit to an old cemetery, especially a rural cemetery, will testify. In the U.S. in 1935, nearly 600 women died for every 100,000 live births. The U.S. maternal mortality rate declined in the 1930s and 1940s and then plummeted from the fifties on. The current maternal mortality rate is fewer than 10 per 100,000 live births.[1] Many advances in medical practice contributed to this decline in maternal mortality: the widespread use of antibiotics and blood transfusions, better management of pregnancy and labor, increases in hospital delivery, and better medical training.[2] These advances, developed in urban medical centers, spread across the nation, as even the most rural and remote areas gained better access to prenatal care.

Only a few generations ago, when pregnancy was a significant risk to the mother, doctors often had to destroy the fetus to save the mother. Today when doctors are faced with a difficult labor, one that threatens the life of the mother, they can turn to a range of medical, delivery, and surgical techniques that protect the mother yet permit live birth. This has significantly changed the status of the fetus. Perhaps the best way to mark this change is to look back at the history of the craniotomy, a destructive operation that represents an extreme example of the mother as patient taking precedence over the fetus as patient.

The use and disappearance of the craniotomy is well documented in the standard textbook, *Williams Obstetrics*. Now in its eighteenth edition, *Williams Obstetrics* was first published in 1903. The first six editions were written by J. Whitridge Williams, the head of the Department of Obstetrics at Johns Hopkins University from 1899 to his death in 1931. The dominant figure in the emergence of modern obstetrics, Williams is reputed to have held a "virtual monopoly" over the appointment of chairs of obstetrics departments in the early twentieth century.[3] From the seventh edition on, new authors revised Williams's original. Their revisions chronicle both continuities and changes in obstetrical practice over this century.[4]

The craniotomy was a simple, if horrifying, procedure. As Williams describes it in the 1903 edition of his text, "Craniotomy usually includes two steps: first, the perforation of the head and the evacuation of its contents; and, secondly, the extraction of the mutilated child."[5] The illustration in Figure 6-1, which accompanies Williams's description, underscores the horror. Although the frequencies varied widely from country to country and between cities and rural areas, craniotomies were not uncommon during the nineteenth century. In 1850s England, one out of every 220 labors ended with craniotomy.[6] Nevertheless, when Williams described the procedure, craniotomy was already in decline, a grotesque reminder of the limits of medical science.

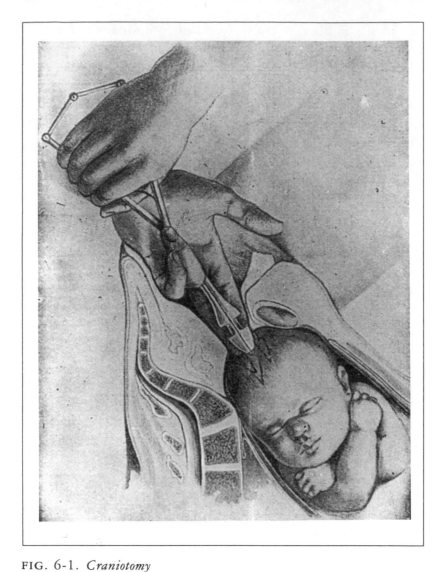

FIG. 6-1. *Craniotomy*

Reprinted by permission from Henricus J. Stander, *Williams Obstetrics: A Textbook for the Use of Students and Practitioners,* 7th edition (New York: D. Appleton-Century Co., 1936), 632.

However, at the turn of the century, craniotomy was still the medically indicated procedure in a range of conditions. If the fetus died in the womb, craniotomy was always indicated if the mother could not easily deliver the stillbirth. Williams warned, "Aesthetic consideration should never deter the operator from resorting to it."[7] Craniotomy was also performed on a live fetus when the fetus's head was too large for the mother's pelvic opening (cephalopelvic disproportion). In 1903, prior to the common practice of cesarean sections,[8] Williams insisted that:

> [A]lthough it must ever be the duty of the obstetrician to do his best to save the life of both mother and child, it is nevertheless readily conceivable that conditions may arise under which craniotomy upon the living child may not only be perfectly justifiable, but even imperatively demanded.[9]

Doctors destroyed the fetus to save the mother because there were few alternatives. In 1878, less than half of the women given cesareans survived. By 1920, mortality was reduced to ten percent, but ten percent mortality is still a risky operation. Moreover, the risks were not evenly distributed, leading Williams to advise, "In country districts, where a physician is unable to summon sufficient assistance, and is without the necessary appliances for an aseptic abdominal operation, Caesarean section should not be undertaken and craniotomy becomes the operation of choice."[10]

At the turn of the century, there were two alternatives to craniotomy that were safer than cesarean. Doctors could either sever the pelvic bone (pubiotomy) or the cartilage connecting the pelvis (symphysiotomy) to enlarge the opening and permit live birth. Both of these operations, especially the second, left many women crippled. In most cases Williams still recommended the craniotomy over these operations.

Thus the mother's health, not just her life, took precedence over the life of the fetus. In later editions of *Williams,* the mother's health was extended to her fertility. In the 1936 edition, the new editor, H. J. Stander, added a new reason for choosing craniotomy over cesarean done late in labor.

> In such circumstances in a primiparous woman [pregnant for the first time] the child should be sacrificed in the interest of the mother, as the only safe alternative consists in cesarean section followed by hysterectomy, which inevitably entails complete abolition of the reproductive function.[11]

Although medically acceptable, craniotomy became the focus of controversy, reflecting concerns about the priority given the mother over the fetus in standard medical practice. At the turn of the century, a minority of doctors and the Catholic Church argued that craniotomy should never be performed. In this view, preventing the death of or injury to the mother never justified killing the near-term fetus. In 1917, the Reverend A. J. Schulte told a gathering of obstetricians that "Better that a million mothers die than one innocent creature be killed."[12] Williams and the subsequent editors of his text rejected that as "too radical a view."[13] The medical establishment continued to insist that the mother was the primary patient.

Although the safety of the cesarean improved in the 1930s, the description of craniotomy in the 1945 edition of *Williams Obstetrics* is remarkably similar to Williams's original. But the 1950 edition marks a complete change.

> Thanks to more widespread prenatal care, the more astute management of pelvic contractions, the availability of sulfonamides and penicillin, and improvements in extraperitoneal cesarean section, craniotomy . . . is never employed today on living infants except in the case of hydrocephalus.[14]

By their very repulsiveness craniotomies demonstrated the medical priority given birthing mothers over the fetus. Doctors were taught to destroy the near-term fetus to save the life, or even preserve the health and fertility, of the woman. This is no longer the case. The elimination of this operation allowed by advances in medical practice helped to define the fetus as a patient.

Advances in fetal medicine and surgery continue to elevate the status of the fetus. As doctors are also better able to monitor fetal development and anticipate problems at birth or with newborns, they are treating the fetus more like a patient. In particular, sonograms have allowed doctors to chart growth and development, enabling them to reassure adults that development is normal or prepare them for problems. Although most current medical practice treats young fetuses as tissue, the image of fetus as patient confers a level of medical personhood that over time may change how doctors treat fetal remains. As Rosalind Petchesky summarizes:

> As one neonatologist told me: "We can do an entire anatomical workup [with a sonogram]!" . . . But the point is that the foetus, through visualization, is being treated as a patient already, it is being given an ordinary check-up. Inference about its "personhood" (or "babyhood") seem verified by sonographic "evidence" that it kicks, spits, excretes, and grows.[15]

More and more fetal health problems can be treated in the womb so that, therapeutically, the woman and her fetus are becoming distinguishable.[16] For example, life-threatening fluid buildups in the fetus's brain or kidney can be treated by surgically inserting a drain. In these operations the fetus is partially removed, placed on the operating table, surgically repaired, and returned to the womb. As these and other operations become safer and more common, they raise the potential conflicts between a "pregnant woman's right to inviolability, autonomy, and treatment refusal, and . . . the unborn child's (at least arguable) rights to prenatal care and life, perhaps including a right to prenatal surgery in some circumstances."[17] Fetal surgery is so new that conflicts over the patient rights of women and fetuses

are rare. More common (but still rare) are the previously discussed medical conflicts over the decision to have a cesarean
delivery.

Some observers foresee a day when pregnancy will involve
two doctors, one for the mother, another for the fetus.[18] Even
though all treatment of the fetus requires going through the
mother—in the case of fetal surgery literally cutting through
the mother—Griener comments that, "In the past, the only way
to affect the fetus' condition was by treating the mother. Now
she can be *bypassed* (emphasis added)."[19] Medical advances raise
new issues about the status of the fetus and the mother. Is the
fetus the patient and the mother merely a container whose
concerns and preferences can be "bypassed" to care for the
fetus?

In most pregnancies the medical needs of the mother and
fetus concur, but in many situations their needs conflict. A fetus
may pose significant risk to a woman with heart or kidney disease. Treating a woman for cancer can threaten her fetus, and,
conversely, treating a fetus either medically or surgically puts
the mother at risk. If the fetus is considered a patient, whose
rights take precedent? Does a fetus have the right to prenatal
care, including the right to surgery? Does the pregnant woman
have the right to deny medical care to her fetus based on her
beliefs and personal fears?

Ironically, being a patient is a peculiar and limited form of
personhood. Critics of modern medicine complain that patients
are dehumanized, that they are treated like bodies or biochemical systems, not people. Robert Hahn, a medical anthropolo-
gist, laments how scientific obstetrics has reduced mothers and
pregnant women to "maternal organisms."[20] But, paradoxically,
illness and modern medicine have enhanced the status of the
fetus. The difference is based on the different initial status.
Defining the fetus as a patient implies some status as a person,
and, however dehumanizing the patient experience, patients are
treated with greater respect than tissue.

7 The Ethics of Fetal Research and the Abortion Conflict

Ambiguities in the definition of the fetus and different perceptions of the fetus have confounded efforts to develop research standards that would be ethically acceptable to opponents of the research. If the young, previable fetus is accorded full status as a person or patient, then the ethical barriers to fetal research are insurmountable, and the only ethical position is to stop all research that does not benefit the participating fetus. This definition may preclude research on dead fetuses as well. As Kathleen Noland insists, "Perfunctory dicing, shearing, pounding—all perfectly acceptable for an excised tumor or kidney—require special justification when the 'tissue fragment' is a fetal corpse."[1]

If, at the other extreme, the fetus is defined as merely maternal tissue, like an excised tumor or kidney, then regardless of whether the tissue is living or dead, the ethical questions evaporate. In this view, the living fetus is not a human research subject nor is the dead fetus a corpse, and research with discarded tissue need not conform to the strict rules of human research ethics.[2] The ethical dilemmas are reduced to the procurement of a "nonessential organ to the scientific community."[3] This perspective frees researchers from ethical constraints. Indeed some argue that the desire to do research encourages scientists to define the fetus as discarded tissue.

Finding some middle ground in the person-versus-tissue debate that permits some research yet satisfies ethical restraints common in human experimentation poses difficult moral and policy judgments. This middle ground is elusive, in part, because of the rapid changes of fetal development and the many forms of fetal research.[4] This middle ground is also a moral and political battlefield because of the dependence of fetal research on planned abortion.

Standards for medical research ethics often come from instances of medical research abuse, many of which were headline news: Nazi experiments on incarcerated Jews, hepatitis studies done with retarded children at Willowbrook Hospital, withholding penicillin to maintain a control group of syphilis patients in Tuskegee, Alabama, injecting live cancer cells into old patients at the Brooklyn Jewish Chronic Disease Hospital, and the recent reports of government-sponsored scientists exposing nonconsenting patients to high doses of radiation in the 1940s and 1950s.

In one of these radiation studies, researchers at Vanderbilt University gave 819 pregnant women a solution containing radioactive iron so they could measure the amount of iron in the women's blood and urine.[5] Three of the 634 children born to the treated women later died of cancer (not all of the treated women gave birth), whereas none of the 655 children born to the untreated women developed childhood cancer. Even though the apparent increase in the cancer rate could, given the small sample, be a coincidence, today such research would be considered too risky except for women planning to have an abortion. While these examples of abuse were made momentarily public, many more abuses occur unbeknownst to the public and are often perpetrated by researchers who gain prominence in their profession.[6]

The tension between the headlong drive for progress and the ethical limits to human experimentation came to the fore this century. World War II was a watershed in modern medicine; many of the advances in antibiotics and surgery, as well as improved treatment of dysentery, malaria, and influenza occurred during the war years. All forms of medical care benefited from these advances; for example, the infant and maternal mortality rates plummeted after the war. Although the grotesque Nazi experiments grabbed postwar headlines as the symbol of research gone mad, the war strained medical ethics in the U.S. as well.[7]

As David Rothman recounts, the war justified taking greater risks with research subjects.[8] Soldiers, institutionalized children and adults, and conscientious objectors were drafted into the war against disease. For example, ten boys at the Cincinnati Children's Hospital were injected with massive doses of dysentery bacteria: all got immediately and severely sick—the average maximum temperature was 104.6 degrees. Although the boys recovered and some developed partial immunity to dysentery, the researchers concluded that their reaction was too severe to be practical as a form of vaccination.[9]

Such research was allowed, even encouraged, because of the belief that "in wartime the effort to conquer disease entitled [medical researchers] to choose martyrs to scientific progress."[10] Although wartime conditions legitimize any number of actions considered immoral in times of peace, the tension between the press of progress and the restraint of ethics is felt each day throughout the research community. This tension pulls especially hard on those engaged in fetal research; they see the promise of such research yet face the accusations of research opponents who compare them to "Nazi scientists torturing helpless babies."

The dispute over fetal research parallels two different approaches to biomedical research ethics. The first relies on absolute standards and assumes that if the research does not comply with specific ethical codes, such as "all research subjects must give informed consent," then the research should not be done, no matter how important. Deciding on and articulating the appropriate standards may require difficult ethical judgments, but once absolute standards are established the ethical dilemmas surrounding specific research projects are simplified: such standards define what research can and cannot be done.

Proponents of absolute standards argue that the scientific gains are not worth the cost in human values from stretching ethics or finding loopholes. Hans Jonas argues that the danger from disease is no less than "the erosion of moral values whose loss, possibly caused by too ruthless a pursuit of scientific progress, would make its most dazzling triumphs not worth having."[11] This approach to biomedical ethics corresponds to the orientation of many abortion and fetal research opponents but is rejected by most scientists.

Opposed to absolute standards, many scientists argue that rigid standards cannot do justice to the difficult trade-offs inherent in medical decisions and that biomedical research ethics require balancing risks and benefits. This second approach requires close scrutiny of the promise, not just the procedures, of the research. If the promised benefits are high, then greater risks to the research subject are justified. And if the risks are slight, then research with only modest potential may be considered worthwhile.[12]

In fetal research, it is difficult to define risk. Most fetal research depends on abortion, and risk is obviously meaningless in research that uses aborted remains. With dead fetuses or fetal tissue, as with a dead person, the problem is one of respect, not risk. This line of reasoning, however, breaks down when extended to the before-abortion fetus. For example, when Dr. Sabath and his colleagues wanted to study the effects of antibiotics on the fetus, they chose to experiment on women planning an abortion rather than those looking forward to a healthy baby. Even if the risk of harm of the medication was slight, they used soon-to-be-aborted fetuses in their experiment rather than take even the slightest risk with wanted fetuses. Abortion became a safety feature of their experiment. To fetal research opponents, the reliance on planned abortion could eliminate restraint, since nearly all research is worth doing when the added risk is zero.

In deciding the balance of risks and benefits, often the interests of patients, the patients' families, and researchers conflict. In biomedical research with fetuses, the question of who decides if the fetus can participate becomes an issue of who can give or withhold proxy consent. Proxy consent assumes that someone can give informed consent for another. Typically a parent or parents are called to give proxy consent for research on, or treatment of, young children, or, at the other end of the life cycle, adult children are asked for their proxy consent on behalf of their incompetent parents.

Proxy consent is not, however, really a form of consent, but rather it is the exercise of authority, presumably legitimate authority, of someone over the life of another. We rely on proxy consent precisely when the consent of the participating individual is not feasible.[13] In a way, when courts interfere and order treatment for a child, they argue that the parents are not fulfilling their obligation to give proxy consent and the state needs to take over this responsibility.

The decision to have an abortion, however, complicates the accepted role of parents in giving consent. Opponents of fetal research argue that once a woman has decided to have an abortion, she is no longer acting in the interest of her fetus; to them the abortion decision voids the accepted right of parents to give proxy consent. Medical ethicist Paul Ramsey summarizes this view by stating that it would be "morally outrageous . . . to designate women who elect abortions for comparatively trivial reasons, or for social convenience or economic betterment," to decide whether or not a fetus will be a research subject.[14]

Moreover, the accepted bases for proxy consent do not apply in fetal research. The parent or guardian asked to give proxy

informed consent is obliged to base that judgment on either
what the research subject would have wanted or on what is in
the subject's best interest.[15] Neither criteria makes sense with
an aborted fetus.

This is all the more troubling to research opponents because
most fetal research is not therapeutic. Therapeutic research is
an experimental treatment that is expected to work but has not
yet been proven safe and effective enough to be considered a
standard treatment. With rare exceptions, none of the fetuses
participating in research will themselves benefit. The exceptions
are the new fetal treatments and surgeries, such as the operation
to correct hydrocephalus.

Viewing research ethics as balancing risks and benefits also
raises the difficult problem of whether or not there is a scientific
imperative; that is, is research, especially medical research, in-
herently beneficial so that we need a good reason to stop it?
The scientific imperative shifts the burden of proof to those
who want to halt or restrain research and away from those who
advocate it.

Part of the scientific imperative is the shift of perspectives
from individual to societal benefit. In many cases, the individuals
participating in highly experimental biomedical research are unlikely to benefit personally; if the research bears fruit, however,
others who did not take the risks may benefit greatly. Taking
social benefit into account changes the risk-benefit calculation
because we weigh individual risk against the potential social
gain of medical progress. Medical researchers think of their
work as a benefit to all, not solely to the patients participating
in the study, and most believe that all knowledge will someday
benefit someone. To researchers, social gain is a necessary factor
in any risk-benefit calculation.

Fetal research, from the routine testing of drugs to the fantastic application of fetal tissue transplants, greatly benefits, or
could greatly benefit, society. We no longer need to wait for
an increase in birth defects to learn of the effects of drugs on

a fetus, surgeons are no longer helpless when a fetus develops some malformations, and fetal tissue may someday rejuvenate damaged or worn-out nerve cells. Many of us, scientists and nonscientists alike, may accept the abstract principle that there is no right to progress, that there is no social obligation that requires medical researchers to develop new cures and treatments.[16]

Nonetheless, suffering, whether from Alzheimer's or AIDS, compels a response. In his essay, "Becoming a Doctor," Lewis Thomas writes of this compulsion to act: "What is it that we expected from our shamans, millennia ago, and still require from the contemporary masters of the [medical] profession? To *do* something, that's what."[17] And, if there is nothing to do—no treatment, no cure—we also feel compelled, however unfairly, to blame researchers and their government sponsors for failing to discover treatments sooner: we want, and increasingly demand, progress. Medical progress even has its own lobby. In a full-page ad in the *New York Times,* Americans for Medical Progress solicited members and contributions "to inform American opinion leaders and citizens about the importance of biomedical research . . . in the quest for new cures."[18] Although ethically questionable, the scientific imperative is, nonetheless, felt by physicians and researchers. It is present both in the hospital wards where doctors are anxious for new treatments and in the labs where scientists dream of discoveries.

Fetal research, in its various forms, severely stretches the standard principles of medical ethics, but it is the link between fetal research and abortion that focused the public spotlight on these ethical problems. Proponents of fetal research insist that abortion and fetal research are, or at least can be made to be, separate issues. They see a clear distinction between family-planning abortions and the other uses of the fetus and fetal tissue.[19]

Those who argue against any moral connection between the two issues often make an analogy to using an organ from someone who was murdered or died in a car crash: clearly using these organs does not condone or even promote murder or reckless driving. Proponents of fetal research reason that whatever the cause of death, death is now a fact or, with a planned abortion, will soon be a fact. If opponents claim that immoral abortion taints fetal research, proponents insist that, right or wrong, abortion exists. In their view it is immoral to waste the opportunity for research, research that may help future fetuses or suffering adults.[20]

Although the decisions to have an abortion and to participate in fetal research are often distinct, fetal research depends on abortion. Without planned abortion, many fetal research projects could not proceed. As will be discussed in detail later, Reagan and Bush administration bans on the funding of fetal tissue transplantation that used aborted tissue effectively halted the research.

A planned abortion allows doctors to create controlled experiments in which specific levels of drugs or other substances can be given to the mother or the fetus. How these drugs are metabolized and what are their specific effects on developing cells and organs can then be detailed in a postabortion autopsy. Planned abortion allows medical researchers to conduct studies that are too risky when no abortion is planned, and to perform them with a level of scientific control that is not possible with spontaneous abortions or retrospective studies of birth defects. Abortion greatly enhances the science while eliminating the need to take risks with wanted fetuses. Furthermore, research relying on abortion increases the safety for other fetuses by providing medical knowledge and improved treatments.

Prenatal diagnosis is also closely associated with abortion on two levels. First, experimental procedures, such as the development of embryoscopy, are first tried on fetuses scheduled for abortion. But, more directly, until medical science develops procedures to correct the problems revealed by prenatal diagnosis, abortion remains the only medical solution. When the prenatal diagnosis is Down's syndrome, anencephaly, or Tay-Sachs disease, the only medical option to delivery of a disabled child is abortion. Advances in fetal therapy and surgery may, in time, add new options, but at present prenatal diagnosis and abortion are closely linked.

Abortion is also necessary for fetal tissue transplants.[21] It is theoretically possible to get tissue for transplant from spontaneous abortions, stillbirths, and ectopic pregnancies; some of the early transplant studies claimed to use such tissue. But tissue from these sources presents major, perhaps insurmountable, problems to researchers. Although approximately 15 to 20 percent of pregnancies end in miscarriages, most early miscarriages occur away from hospitals or clinics, greatly complicating tissue recovery. In late miscarriages and stillbirths, the fetus has most often died weeks earlier, rendering the tissue useless for study or transplantation.

Moreover, doctors believe that most spontaneous abortions are the result of fetal abnormalities; for example, chromosomal deformities exist in 60 percent of first-trimester miscariages.[22] With such high rates of abnormalities, researchers must assume that tissue from miscarriages is unhealthy. It must be cultured, examined, and proven healthy before it can be used in research and therapy. By the time tissue health is determined, the tissue may no longer be useful to science or for transplantation.

Another potential source of fetal tissue is animals; an issue that is controversial in itself.[23] At this time, most fetal tissue transplantation research has relied on animals; primarily lab rats The question at this stage is not what is the role of lab animals in research but should nonhuman fetal tissue be used for transplantation into humans. While some surgeons are experimenting with transplanting baboon organs into humans, researchers are wondering if large, nonhuman primates could become fetal tissue donors. Many of these primates are themselves endangered species, and many scientists question the ethics, as well as the practicality, of using them in research. They ask, how can we justify killing endangered primates that "are scarce, expensive, hard to breed, and not a totally satisfactory analogue" when aborted fetuses are readily available.[24]

In contrast to miscarriages, elective abortion allows physicians to plan to receive and preserve the fetal tissue. Even though most abortions stop fetal life signs and dismember the fetus, abortion produces fresher and more intact tissue than do miscarriages. Moreover, legal elective abortion means that fetal tissue is abundant and readily available, two crucial issues if fetal tissue transplants ever become standard practice. Thus, fetal research, and the procuring of tissue and organs from fetuses, are procedurally, if not morally, linked to elective abortion. Fetal research in general and fetal tissue transplantation in particular could not continue without abortion.

The needs of research may also change abortion practice. Some forms of abortion, such as hysterotomies, yield fetuses better suited for research and tissue donation than other forms. Abortion by hysterotomy involves the surgical removal of the intact fetus; in some cases, as alleged in the hysterotomy that led to Dr. Edelin's arrest, the aborted fetus can show some fleeting life signs. Hysterotomies are generally performed in the second trimester, when the fetus is quite developed, and they are the most controversial form of abortion; from the mid-1950s to the early 1970s they were common, but now they are extremely rare.

Some fear that progress in fetal tissue transplantation may lead us to the point where the need for certain types of tissue— more intact tissue from more developed fetuses—will put pressure on women to opt for a hysterotomy. While it is unlikely that hysterotomies will once again become common in the developed world, poor women living in impoverished countries may become easy targets for tissue markets.

Even if research needs do not increase the rate of hysterotomies, they may encourage minor changes in abortion practices, changes that do not significantly increase the risk or discomfort to the woman patient. Rather than the singular concern for a safe and trouble-free abortion, research needs may encourage doctors to try to better preserve and recover fetal tissue. For example, doctors could use ultrasound to locate the fetus prior to abortion and then use clear, detachable suction tubes to help separate fetal tissue from other tissue during the abortion.[25]

Fetal research could also alter the timing of an abortion. In studies of how little, and how much, common medications cross the placenta, researchers may ask a pregnant woman to delay her abortion a day or two, or to come in for the experimental treatment a day or two prior to her abortion, to facilitate the experiment. Research opponents worry that participating in an experiment that poses even slight risk to the fetus could discourage a woman from changing her mind about the abortion. And if more mature tissue proves especially valuable for transplantation, women could be pressured into delaying abortion. Older fetuses yield more tissue, and tissue at a higher level of functional maturity may prove better for some transplantation.[26]

In addition to these procedural connections between fetal research and abortion, opponents fear that fetal research and life-restoring fetal transplants will legitimize abortion, acting as an indirect incentive—or weaken the disincentives—for abortion. The possible social benefit that could come from participation in research may persuade some undecided women to choose abortion. What they dread most, however, is the possibility that a woman would actually become pregnant to abort and provide tissue for research or treatment.

Opponents also argue that the use of aborted fetuses taints the subsequent uses of fetal tissue, much like the Nazi experiments tainted the use of their research findings. Researchers using fetal tissue may not know the source and may have had nothing to do with the abortion decision: they merely receive the tissue from a supplier much like a surgeon would receive a donated organ. To the opponents of abortion, however, fetal research is part of an immoral conspiracy, and researchers are, in their view, accomplices to murder.[27] Thus, a significant and active group of citizens see fetal research and abortion as connected. In the view of the antiabortion movement, fetal research is one more way the fetus is immorally abused.

Fetal research comes in many forms: some fetal research, like ultrasound measurements, is so routine and noninvasive that it raises few ethical concerns, whereas other research—especially fetal tissue transplants—stretches both medical knowledge and ethics. The status of the fetus in law, medical practice, and among different groups in our society is ambiguous and changing. Different factions cannot agree if a fetus is a person, when it becomes a person, and what ethical principles apply at various stages of development and in various forms of research. These basic ambiguities are the foundation of the protracted social and political struggle over fetal research.

There are no technical or ethical solutions for these dilemmas, and the association of fetal research with abortion—a practical association founded in the research protocols and a moral association felt by abortion opponents—thrusts these most difficult issues into the political arena. Proponents of fetal research cannot abandon what they consider as an important and promising area of research. They cannot foreclose the possibility of medical advances just because opponents have raised unresolved and, perhaps, unresolvable ethical dilemmas. On the other hand, opponents of fetal research will not accept the compromises designed to assuage their moral concern. They cannot conclude that if the rules are followed, then the research can go on.

8 The First Legislation

Congress and the Fetal Research Controversy

In May 1973, one month after the first protest at the National Institutes of Health, Angelo Roncallo, a Right-to-Life Republican congressman from New York, proposed the first ban on fetal research. Responding to stories of fetuses being kept alive in tanks and experiments on severed fetal heads, Roncallo's ban prohibited Health, Education, and Welfare, NIH's parent department, from funding "research in the United States or abroad on a human fetus while it is outside the uterus of its mother and which has a beating heart."[1] This amendment to the National Biomedical and Behavioral Research Training program defined the nonviable fetus outside the womb as a born person, and if its heart beats, a living person. It passed the House of Representatives by a vote of 354 to 9. A similar, easily passed amendment prohibited the National Science Foundation from funding live fetus research, even though NSF never funded such research.

These first congressional bans on fetal research quickly became part of a larger debate on the ethics of human experimentation. Revelations of ethical abuses, such as the Tuskegee Syphilis Studies, had sparked congressional concern, with Senator Ted Kennedy holding hearings on research ethics and sponsoring legislation to more closely regulate biomedical research. The hearings, held prior to the April 1973 protests, covered a wide range of issues, from psychosurgery to drug trials, but fetal research was never discussed. The protests of April brought this issue out of the shadows just as Senator Kennedy was shepherding his medical ethics bill through Congress. Fetal research became the subject of legislative debate by historical coincidence.

On September 11, 1973, Senator James Buckley, the brother of *Firing Line* host Bill Buckley, proposed an amendment to Kennedy's bill that would permanently ban much fetal research. His amendment states:

> The Secretary [of HEW] may not conduct or support research or experimentation in the United States or abroad, whether before or after induced abortion, unless such research or experimentation is done for the purpose of insuring the survival of that fetus or infant.[2]

This ban has several important differences from Roncallo's. First, it is more extensive. It precludes all nontherapeutic research, not just live-fetus research. Second, it explicitly links the ban to abortion: the same research that would be outlawed by this ban would be approved were it not for the abortion connection.

The inclusive phrase "before or after abortion" proved especially troubling to research supporters, since they could not be certain if a woman's decision to have an abortion after participating in research would violate the ban. The ban would prohibit fetal researchers from using abortion to increase scientific control and reduce risk to other, wanted fetuses. To fetal research opponents, abortion changes the ethical context; anything associated with abortion is wrong. In their view, fetal research must start from the premise—a premise not shared by most researchers—that the fetus is a person, not tissue or a lab animal. Buckley told the Senate that "my amendment is predicated on the fact that . . . a human fetus is in fact a human fetus."[3]

Kennedy was sympathetic to the moral arguments of his more stridently Right-to-Life Senate colleague. His Catholicism and his concern for biomedical ethics created much common ground between this liberal senator and the staunchly conservative Buckley. He shared Buckley's outrage at the press accounts of experiments on living fetuses but was also worried that the ban would halt medical progress. "Part of the problem that is suggested by the amendment of the Senator from New York [Buckley] is its restrictive nature," Kennedy said in a floor speech. "Scientists are on the verge of some important breakthroughs. . . . So I would like to ask my friend from New York if he is not concerned by the limitations of the possibilities for research . . . which offer a very great opportunity to try to provide relief for children yet unborn. . . ."[4]

Of course, scientists are always on the verge of breakthroughs. Nonetheless, Kennedy worried that banning nontherapeutic research that relied on abortion would impede progress, a view championed by scientists. Buckley, on the other hand, merely dismissed the dilemma, saying that his amendment would halt only unethical research and that progress would not be endangered.[5] Others in the Senate also felt that the ban would impede progress but they, like Kennedy, wanted it both ways.

Wanting progress but also wanting to restrain some of the research that begets progress, Kennedy proposed and won support (by a 53-to-35 vote) for a "perfecting amendment" to Buckley's ban. Kennedy accepted this "before and after abortion" ban but added language to make it temporary. His ethics bill already proposed creating the National Commission for the Protection of Human Subjects,[6] and he now assigned them the task of examining fetal research. Unable to resolve congressional ambivalence about fetal research, the bill, setting a precedent for this and future disputes over science, entrusted the controversy to an expert panel.

On June 6, 1974, after struggling over the composition, term, and responsibilities of the National Commission, Congress passed and President Nixon signed the National Research Act.[7] The law lauded science's many contributions and reaffirmed the nation's support for research. Nevertheless, it temporarily banned nontherapeutic fetal research; this one area of research would no longer receive federal support.

After the passage of the 1974 National Research Act, the fetal research controversy shifted venue from Congress to the bureaucracy, where HEW and the National Commission struggled to find a resolution. Congress did not lose interest in abortion, however. Having lost in the Supreme Court, abortion opponents tried new tactics to outlaw abortion. Throughout the early to mid-1970s, Right-to-Life organizations worked to elect antiabortion legislators and to hold those elected to the rigid, "either for or against abortion" discipline of single-interest politics.[8]

During this period, antiabortionists tried to pass two bills which would overturn *Roe* v. *Wade*.[9] The first was the Right-to-Life Amendment to the Constitution, which, if ratified, would give a fetus full citizenship rights from the moment of conception. When this most restrictive amendment failed to get the necessary two-thirds support in Congress, antiabortion legislators tried to pass the Human Life Bill. Although it lacked the symbolic clout of a constitutional amendment, this bill, if passed, would have granted the newly fertilized embryo Fourteenth Amendment equal rights protection.

If either the amendment or the bill had passed, nontherapeutic fetal research would be halted forever; Buckley's amendment would, in effect, be made permanent. In research, as in all other matters, the embryo and fetus would be granted equal status to adults and children, and, since proxy consent is dubious for a fetus being considered for nontherapeutic research or an abortion, all such research would stop. Halting such research was, of course, one reason antiabortionists proposed the laws. In the words of one supporter of these bills, "By repudiating *Roe* and renewing the Constitution's commitment to life, the amendment will end the 'hunt, destroy, and experiment' syndrome that has turned some scientific researchers from protectors of human life to exploiters of human life."[10]

By 1980, Right-to-Life groups helped put Ronald Reagan in the White House and expand the antiabortion voting block in Congress. Reagan, however, jilted the new right–antiabortion coalition by failing to push the Right-to-Life Amendment and the Human Life Bill, which were then abandoned in the early 1980s. Despite its most graphic appeals for support—one Life Amendment Political Action Committee mailing featured photos of dead fetuses[11]—the public and, therefore, most legislators were not willing to extend citizenship rights to a newly fertilized egg. They were not willing to resolve by fiat the legal and social ambiguities surrounding the fetus.

During this period, controversy over fetal research was not restricted to Washington, D.C.; it spread to state capitals across the country. Prior to *Roe* v. *Wade*, many state antiabortion laws also regulated the uses of aborted fetuses, and therefore fetal research. In the months after *Roe*, four states—California, Indiana, Minnesota, and South Dakota— passed restrictive fetal research laws, and in 1974 five states and in 1976 two more states followed suit. By the mid-1980s, twenty-five states passed laws explicitly regulating fetal research.[12]

Many of these state laws are only symbolic: for example, even though Wyoming and Montana passed antifetal research legislation, neither state has labs set up to perform the research in the first place. Laws in states that are centers of biomedical research, such as California and Massachusetts, have serious implications for fetal research, however. In these states, the dispute over state laws and regulations portray the fetal research conflict in miniature.

In the early 1970s, William Delahunt was elected to the Massachusetts House of Representatives with the support of Right-to-Life groups, who, once in office, brought fetal research to his attention.[13] Antiabortionists repeated to Delahunt the now familiar litany of grotesque research that had first sparked public protest—live fetuses in tanks, severed fetal heads, jabbing needles into the soon-to-be-aborted—convincing him of the need for regulation. With the help of James Smith, a professor at the Jesuit Boston College Law School, he wrote a bill that banned all research on fetuses, whether living or dead, before or after abortion.

In the statehouse the bill faced little resistance until researchers from the Harvard Medical School spoke up for their research. After learning of a hearing scheduled for the next day, Harvard's dean for clinical affairs, Jack Ewalt, started calling experts, most of whom claimed that they were too busy to get involved. At the hearing, Ewalt presented letters from Nobel laureates and the testimony of one lone fetal researcher, and Delahunt decided to set up a meeting with researchers to work out their differences. Like many legislators, Delahunt was against abortion but for research; he also wanted it both ways.

This group drafted compromise language that would allow research on the then-experimental amniocentesis and studies of fetal tissue. Nevertheless the compromise would still have prohibited much fetal research, such as the work of David Nathan, who was refining fetal blood-sampling techniques for detecting genetic hemoglobin disorders. He was convinced that his research was both important and moral; if proven safe, fetal blood tests could reduce the need for abortion for women who learned that their fetus was healthy despite the risks of an inherited disease such as Tay-Sachs or sickle-cell anemia. He presented his case to the committee but did not like the compromise. "I was in a rage, I felt we were selling out."[14]

Nathan, among others, lobbied hard for changes in the bill. He complained that the bill would slow medical progress, that he and others were close to major advances in prenatal diagnosis. This argument rang a resonant cord, even among Right-to-Life legislators such as Delahunt, but restriction supporters were still concerned about the connection between fetal research and abortion. The bill was revised to clarify the consent process so that it separated the research and the abortion decisions but still prohibited research on fetuses scheduled for abortion, like Nathan's blood-sampling studies.

The final result of the Massachusetts controversy was a law that significantly restricts nontherapeutic fetal research in a state that is a center for biomedical research. That the law does not ban all fetal research outright is the result of the efforts of scientists to convince elected officials of the importance of their research. The scientists were partially successful in presenting their case, but the very engagement infuriated many scientists who do not feel the need to justify their work to politicians, especially state politicians who do not fund their research. The Harvard scientists resented the need to plead their case, to go to the statehouse and ask, "Please, Mr. Legislator, may I go on with what I am doing?"[15] The ban and the need to dirty their hands with politics was, for them, a loss of autonomy.

Back in Washington, after the first storm of protest in April 1973, HEW took the first tentative steps toward resolving the conflict. Building on the work of the 1971 NIH study group, HEW in November 1973 proposed a new set of research guidelines.[16] Despite concern that openness might prolong the controversy, Robert Stone, then director of NIH, hoped that public scrutiny of the department's proposals might help resolve the issues.

These new guidelines focused directly on issues raised by Right-to-Life groups. They restated the importance of parental consent in therapeutic research but concluded that consent is insufficient when there is no potential benefit to the participating fetus. Research relying on abortion falls into this category, since the fetus is not expected to survive. HEW also proposed establishing an ethics advisory board at the federal level. Delegating questions of social benefit and ethical standards to this advisory board would limit the authority of the local institutional review boards that monitored research practice. HEW suggested that only one-third of the ethics advisory board should be scientists; they felt that broader participation would give decisions greater legitimacy.

Thus while sustaining the importance of fetal research, the proposed guidelines attempted to protect its socially acceptable forms. Borrowing language from abortion opponents, HEW concluded that the "respect for the dignity of human life must not be compromised whatever the age, circumstances, or expectation of life of the individuals."[17] Perhaps most important, the proposed guidelines concluded that social values, not scientific merit, are the ultimate criteria in choosing whether to proceed with research or ban it. This point, however, avoids the central feature of controversies over science. The controversy over fetal research testifies to the different values that coexist in our society. Most scientists, for example, consider advancing knowledge and medical practice as a moral, not just technical, goal.

In August 1974, HEW revised its proposal by weakening the research restrictions. The most important aspect of this revision was the large volume of public comment considered: more than 450 responses were sent to HEW regarding the proposals.[18] The overwhelming majority of responses came from scientific organizations who found the guidelines too restrictive. The influence of the scientists was apparent in the next revisions, which now allowed two types of controversial experiments that the draft rules had banned: research that relied on abortion and experiments that sustained the vital life signs, like the controversial artificial placenta studies, were both permitted if the ultimate goal was the refinement of health-care procedures.

This second draft could, depending on how broadly interpreted, include all the controversial studies. Scientists had argued throughout that all fetal research contributed to improved health care. These draft guidelines were remarkably similar to the 1971 NIH study panel recommendations, evidence of the inertia of bureaucratic decisions.

The influence of scientists on these revisions also underscores an important characteristic of disputes over science. Those opposing research express their dissent not through established administrative channels but through public demonstrations, the media, and elected officials. In contrast, scientists avoid the spotlight and prefer to work with administrative agencies, especially those such as NIH that are dominated by scientists. Scientists outside government share the same values and ways of thinking as the professionals and experts that work in the science bureaucracies, and once these agencies are charged with resolving controversies over science, scientists gain the upper hand.

The controversy was far from over, however. The creation and deliberation of the National Commission delayed the approval of the final guidelines one year. Dr. Kenneth Ryan was elected commission chair. He was the head of Harvard's Obstetrics and Gynecology Department and had represented Harvard in negotiations with Massachusetts legislators over the state fetal research ban. Once formed, the commission sponsored studies of the scope of fetal research and the operation of institutional review boards, sampled public opinion in open hearings, and debated the difficult issues.

The report of the commission was similar to HEW's revised guidelines, suggesting once again the inertia of past decisions.[19] They allowed minimal risk, therapeutic research, and called for the strict procedural separation of abortion and research. The commission, like HEW, recommended the creation of a federal ethics advisory board (EAB) to consider case-by-case waivers for nontherapeutic research.

The commission recommendations differed from HEW's on the treatment of the nonviable fetus, however. To avoid confusion in the case of the nonviable fetus when abortion might legitimate risky procedures, the commission defined the nonviable fetus as a dying individual and concluded that no research may use such subjects. In their view, the dignity of the dying was more important than the scientific potential of the research. On this issue they agreed with fetal research critics that an unencumbered death is a human right that overrides the social benefit of medical progress.

Given the difficulty of the issues addressed, the eleven-member commission—three were physicians, three were research scientists, three were lawyers, one was a philosopher, and one a social activist—achieved near consensus on all issues. One commissioner, David Louisell, a law professor, voiced dissent after the recommendations were made public. He agreed with all but one recommendation, the waiver provision that authorized the EAB to balance social benefit against individual rights. Louisell wrote:

> I am compelled to disagree with the Commission's recommendations . . . insofar as they succumb to the error of sacrificing the interests of innocent human life to a postulated social need. . . . Although the Commission uses adroit language, . . . no facile verbal formula can avoid the reality that under these recommendations the fetus and nonviable infant will be subjected to research from which other humans are protected.[20]

With the exception of Louisell, commissioners could not put aside the value of the knowledge promised by nontherapeutic fetal research; they, like HEW and the NIH study group before them, felt a need to forge a solution, if only by adroit language, that allowed most research to continue.

But even the absolute ban on research on the dying fetus proved too restrictive for HEW. Caspar Weinberger, then HEW secretary, concluded that research designed to enable fetuses to survive must continue. He reasoned that the success of past experiments and the public interest in better health care for premature infants justified including dying fetuses in research. He did not believe that the individual rights of the dying fetus should be allowed to impede medical progress. On July 29, 1975, this final draft was approved and became the regulations governing all fetal research funded by the federal government. The temporary "before and after abortion" ban was lifted.

In 1978, a research team from the Charles R. Drew Postgraduate Medical School submitted a proposal to study the safety of fetal blood sampling guided by an experimental fetoscope. Genetic diagnostic techniques, such as amniocentesis, can identify only a limited number of fetal abnormalities. The blood samples would enable doctors to identify such disabilities as sickle-cell anemia while the fetus is still in the womb. This proposal required approval of the new EAB because the research involved fetuses scheduled for abortion and unknown risk. Fetal blood sampling was, at that time, considered one of the more promising developments in prenatal diagnosis, but doctors were concerned about the risk to the fetus of even small amounts of bleeding.

This was the first, and as it turned out the only, fetal research study reviewed by the EAB.[21] Since the research relied on abortion the EAB had to decide whether or not to apply the "equality maxim," the rule that no research should be done on a fetus scheduled for abortion that would not be done on one expected to go full term. The EAB agreed with research proponents, that biomedical information was in this case too important to prohibit because of the research's reliance on abortion. They approved the specific study and recommended that the secretary of HEW grant a blanket waiver to all fetal blood sampling studies. The only restriction imposed was that the research not alter the timing of the abortion. The research was funded, but HEW secretary Califano did not grant the general exception.[22]

For fetal researchers this decision represents the high point of compromise. Carefully crafted regulations were in place and the EAB made a case-by-case review of studies that violated the general guidelines. When forced to balance the promise of medical breakthroughs against ethical concerns of relying on abortion, the EAB was persuaded by the need for progress; they agreed with researchers in deciding the fate of fetal research that medical benefits outweighed ethical costs.

But to research opponents this decision underscored how abandoning absolutes, such as no research should be done on a fetus before or after an abortion, is quickly translated into a license to do all research. When the issue is framed as balancing costs and benefits, progress always tips the scales for research. Shortly after the fetal blood sampling decision, however, this initial resolution to the fetal research controversy collapsed.

9 The Reagan Years

The Political Standoff Between Supporters

and Opponents of Fetal Research

In 1980, NIH approved a second fetal blood sampling study.[1] Like the earlier one, this study was designed to test prenatal diagnosis of genetic blood diseases[2] and, like the earlier one, relied on abortion to reduce risk to fetuses scheduled to go to full term. This research also required EAB approval, a process expected to be pro forma since the EAB had earlier suggested a blanket approval for all such studies. Approval was, however, no longer possible.

The initial three-year charter for the EAB expired on September 30, 1980, a few days before the Carter-Reagan presidential election. HEW secretary Patricia Harris simply allowed the charter to lapse.[3] Perhaps she thought reconstituting the EAB should be left to the next administration, or perhaps this decision was merely lost in the flurry of the election season. Whatever the reason, this oversight effectively vetoed the compromise crafted five years earlier by the National Commission.[4]

Ronald Reagan won the 1980 election, in part because of the

new right–antiabortion coalition. Although Reagan never pushed antiabortion legislation, especially the constitutional amendments, with the fervor expected by Right-to-Lifers, he did make antiabortion views an essential job requirement for political appointees.

After the 1980 election, these antiabortion appointees looked for any vehicle to eliminate involvement of the federal government in abortion. Eventually they would disallow federal abortion funding for welfare recipients and in military hospitals. These antiabortion administrators never proposed reinstating the EAB, and thus the second fetal blood study was not funded. After 1980, no fetal research that exceeded the minimal-risk standard or that relied on abortion received federal money. As Michell Globus, the principle investigator for the second fetoscopy study lamented, research on the prenatal diagnosis of blood disorders was, from 1980 on, "seriously restricted."[5]

From 1980 until 1988, the fetal research controversy became highly ritualized. In 1982, Representative William Dannemeyer (Republican, California) introduced an amendment to the National Institutes of Health Reauthorization Bill (HR 6357) that, in his words, was "almost identical in form" to the 1973 Buckley amendment restricting fetal research.[6] The Dannemeyer amendment banned all federally sponsored research "on a living fetus or infant, whether before or after induced abortion, unless such research or experimentation is done for the purpose of ensuring the survival of the fetus or infant."[7] Without the EAB to grant exceptions, such research was already disallowed by the current regulations.

Supporters of the amendment again insisted that fetal research compounds the moral outrage of abortion and that pregnant women who have chosen abortion have abdicated their parental right to approve research affecting the fetus. They once again conjured up images of Nazi-like experiments on the helpless to support their opposition to fetal research. As Representative Robert Dornan (Republican, California) argued in the

House debate, "We have sick, very sick, mentally disturbed doctors, an infinitesimal percentage to be sure, that specialize in nothing but the destruction of human life. Then to assuage their consciences they look forward to doing research on living fetuses."[8]

Supporters of the research argued that the amendment addressed a nonexistent problem—that no grotesque experiments had been performed under the existing regulations—and that the vagueness of the wording could stop all fetal research. They saw the amendment as an ideological assault on science, or, as Representative Les AuCoin (Democrat, Oregon) labeled it, "another fever swamp kind of amendment."[9] Representative Henry Waxman (Democrat, California) raised the flag of progress: "this amendment . . . would do a tremendous amount of harm for saving lives, for allowing births to go forward, for allowing babies to mature, and it would lead to ignorance. Ignorance in biomedical research could mean that we are not going to know how to save lives and how to allow a fetus to mature."[10]

Despite these pleas, the Dannemeyer amendment passed the House of Representatives with 260 to 140 votes; however, the NIH reauthorization bill never came to a vote in the Senate, and the amendment never became law. (NIH funding was sustained throughout this stalemate by means of continuing resolutions.) Representative Dannemeyer then attached a slightly reworded amendment to the 1983 NIH reauthorization bill (HR 2350). To counter this amendment, Representative Waxman proposed a substitute that, in effect, wrote the current administrative rules into law. But yet again the amended reauthorization bill was withdrawn before it was voted up or down in Congress.

Delayed for two years by this ritualized confrontation, the Health Research Extension Act (PL 99-158) finally passed in 1985. This law extended NIH funding for three years and restated the 1975 administrative rules regulating fetal research. The law prohibits research on the nonviable fetus unless the research "will pose no additional risk, injury, or death to the fetus and the purpose of the research or experimentation is the development of important biomedical knowledge which cannot be obtained by other means."[11] Medical researchers had insisted throughout the conflict that all fetal research contributes to biomedical knowledge and poses no added risk when abortion is planned. By restating the "social benefit" exemption to the ban on fetal research, the law could have allowed the controversial research to continue.

Antiabortion activists in Congress and the White House nonetheless were able to stop federal funding by exploiting a new procedure established by the 1985 law. This law established a Congressional Biomedical Advisory Board to replace the now-defunct EAB. This board was far more political than the expert panel it replaced. Its members were not researchers and ethicists but twelve members of Congress from both political parties. The board was charged with assembling a fourteen-member committee to, among other things, oversee the granting of waivers to the general ban on nontherapeutic fetal research.

This second-level review committee was not constituted until near the end of the three-year reauthorization, and it never functioned as a review committee. The congressional board spent the time arguing over the abortion views of the prospective members. Supporters and opponents of fetal research wanted assurance that neither could gain a majority. The first National Commission and the EAB were established to remove political wrangling from decisions over fetal research but by the mid-1980s fetal research was inescapably political. Rather than a solution, the congressional board became a further expression of the essential stalemate that had ensnared fetal research.

Exasperating supporters and opponents alike, the political drama over fetal research was, for the decade of the 1980s, just an endless recitation of now-hackneyed arguments. This prolonged controversy did, however, set a stage upon which the clash of values was acted out. Supporters and opponents approached and considered the issues raised from markedly different worldviews, with stands on abortion serving as a "values switch": if you knew someone's stand on abortion, you knew, with near certainty, their views on fetal research.[12] These differences are far greater than the two cultures of science and humanities first described by C. P. Snow[13]; the fetal research dispute is a conflict over the pre-eminence of progress itself.

On this political stage, research supporters reiterate that progress is essential and good; it is valued for itself. This is especially true in medical science. Supporters of fetal research argue that we have a moral obligation to develop new cures, and that it is immoral to waste any opportunity, such as the opportunity provided by abortion, to advance medical science. If scientific progress is a moral imperative, then restraining science is not just an inconvenience; it is wrong. As John Fletcher, a prominent bioethicist, told a congressional hearing, "When viewed by its consequences the moratorium [on fetal research] and the pattern that continues can fairly be called a policy of moral recklessness in the face of great undeserved human suffering."[14]

To reinforce the value of progress, supporters of research repeatedly make the polio analogy. Fetal tissue cultures played a minor and, in all likelihood, a nonessential role in developing the vaccines that ended the polio pandemic. Nevertheless, research supporters recall the frightening disease and the life-saving vaccines because they provide a morality play of scientific progress. No matter how unsettling the constant push of progress may be, no one wants to return to the time when polio crippled so many.

The inherent value of progress is also an expression of national pride. Research supporters argued throughout that it was not enough for the research to be done but that it should be done in the U.S. Even though abortion is uniquely controversial in the U.S., it is important, in their view, that American researchers retain their status as world leaders in biomedicine. Banning fetal research could reduce American scientists to the lowly status of borrowers, rather than creators, of discovery. This is more than an insult to nationalism but a failure of our self-perceived role as world cultural leaders; it is the Vietnam syndrome applied to science.

Because of the inherent value of progress, scientists take a utilitarian approach to dealing with conflicts. They believe in the rational process of balancing risk against gain. To halt research or a new technology simply because there are physical risks or moral costs is, to scientists, irrational because it addresses only one side of the equation.

The metaphor of the scale, of balancing pros and cons, guides research supporters through the difficult moral thickets that surround fetal research. They acknowledge the moral issues raised by research opponents but time and again counterbalance them with actual and anticipated benefits. Opponents argue that scientists tilt the scale by improperly balancing social benefit against individual loss, especially the difficult to define loss of a fetus, and by using abortion to minimize risk. But to scientists, policy decisions should be rational, not absolute.

During this conflict scientists and research supporters also expressed their devotion to research freedom. Bans, even if just funding bans, are described as a threat to intellectual freedom. Though nearly all courts have upheld the government's right to regulate research, research is often equated with protected speech. Research supporters conjure up images of the Spanish Inquisition when dissent was crushed by the church. The stories of Galileo being forced to recant the heliocentric view of the universe, of Nazis labeling Einstein's theories as decadent, and of Stalin compelling biologists to follow Lysenko's, rather than Mendel's, theories of genetics are repeated to warn against the intrusion of politics in science.

These warnings carry a double threat. Political intrusion threatens freedom—the American Civil Liberties Union wrote Congress to protest fetal research bans, arguing that "ideological control over science and medicine is profoundly threatening to a democratic society."[15] The intrusion also threatens progress since, as these examples show, the ideological control postponed scientific and technical advance.

During the conflict, scientists also expressed the view that science policy making must be rooted in technical understanding and, therefore, should be left to the experts. In this view, science policy is different from other government decisions and cannot be trusted to nonexpert politicians or citizens. Even while criticizing fetal research, Peter McCullagh, a scientist, states this bias: "[T]he validity and relevance [of ethical analysis] will remain entirely at the mercy of the biological data which has been used in framing it."[16] Since, in the view of many scientists, ethical arguments are framed by and subservient to technical distinctions, only scientists should participate in decisions about research because only they fully understand the issues. They dismiss research opponents as ideologues.

The singular importance of expertise is also seen in the distinctions made and language used. Scientists base ethical judgments on scientifically observable differences. For example, a viable fetus warrants different treatment from a nonviable one because of observable developmental differences. Advocates of the brain-alive theory struggled mightily, though in vain, to define the moment of life based on clear-cut biological indicators. Scientists also speak a more technical language. They differentiate embryos from fetuses and refer to the fetus *in* and *ex utero*.

In contrast, fetal research opponents use an entirely different language. They do not differentiate an embryo from a fetus but speak of the "unborn." They describe the procurement of fetal tissue as "harvesting babies" and planned abortion as murder. This language is more metaphorical than technical; it expresses their values and political goals. Time and again the words chosen by fetal research opponents simultaneously confer personhood to the fetus—an unborn child is metaphorically more a person than is a nonviable fetus *in utero*—and challenge the authority granted experts by the use of technical jargon. By rejecting their terms, fetal research opponents assert that they have equal status as the scientists in making decisions about fetal research.

Fetal research opponents also reject the cost-benefit reasoning behind most efforts to find compromise. For them the issue is one of right and wrong, not trying to find a gray middle ground that balances the right of medical progress against the wrong of abortion. The very act of accepting a compromise means, to opponents, abandoning the fundamental moral principle—abortion is murder—that forms the basis of their position. This rejection of the form of reasoning behind the efforts to craft a compromise is enormously frustrating to research supporters; opponents will not budge.

Fetal research opponents also draw unflattering portraits of scientists. They are presented as an elite who do not understand commonsense morals. Rather than unworldly geniuses or disinterested experts, research foes often describe researchers as self-serving and career-oriented: in this uncomplimentary portrayal, fetal researchers do their experiments, not for the good of society, but exclusively for their own prestige and profit.

More darkly, opponents commonly refer to fetal researchers as Nazi scientists who, after denying the humanity of the fetus, inflict grotesque experiments on it to satisfy their own demented curiosity. Representative Dannemeyer repeatedly charged doctors of doing research on aborted fetuses to wash away the sin of murder by providing health-giving cures.

As they compare scientists to Nazi doctors, antiabortionists commonly compare themselves to abolitionists. Antiabortionists often compare *Roe* v. *Wade* to the nineteenth-century Dred Scott case, which upheld the right to own slaves. These comparisons have multiple meanings. Right-to-Lifers are culturally similar to the uncompromising and vehement abolitionists, but they are also suggesting that, even if they are currently a minority, history will prove them the champions of human values. Fetal researchers who use aborted fetuses will, by analogy, be seen as the slave owners who allowed self-interest to rationalize immoral views.

Except for the two years of the EAB's brief life, the federal funding ban halted much basic fetal research. Efforts to find a compromise were mired in stalemate. The federal government continued to fund therapeutic, minimal-risk research, and private money provided support for some nontherapeutic research, such as the safety testing of chorionic villus sampling.[17] Studies of human fetal blood sampling all but stopped. This stalemate was, however, soon to be tested by a new form of fetal research: fetal tissue transplantation.

10 New Fetal Tissue Transplant Research, Old Political Controversy

C ontroversy and federal restrictions slowed, but did not halt, fetal research, and in the mid-1980s a new form of research, fetal tissue transplants, was about to spill out of the lab and renew the now-fading controversy. For years, scientists had experimented with fetal tissue transplants in lab animals, and the first, unsuccessful human fetal transplants were tried in the 1920s. During the 1970s animal research proceeded apace, convincing some physicians that it was again time to try the operation on people.

Those interested in fetal tissue transplants recognized that many details must be painstakingly worked out with human trials before the operations could become standard practice. Researchers need to identify the amounts, age, and type of fetal tissue needed; the exact site for the various transplants; the transplantation procedures; and the types of diseases and patients that could be treated. Like any new surgical procedure, fetal tissue transplants would require much trial and error.

In the U.S. a few researchers, such as Drs. Eugene Redman at Yale and Curt Freed at the University of Colorado, began, quietly and warily, to try human fetal tissue transplants. Fetal tissue transplants did not, however, receive the same amount of research attention in the U.S. as they did abroad. The years of controversy had made American researchers cautious; few were willing to attempt research, however promising, that could lead to protest, indictment, or layer upon layer of bureaucratic review. But around the world fetal tissue transplantation became more common.

In the 1980s, Chinese and Soviet[1] surgeons transplanted fetal pancreas tissue into nearly 300 diabetics. Skeptics doubt the value of these operations; results are rarely reported in medical journals and the few published accounts provide inadequate information on procedures and measures of success. (One concern is that success is likely to be reported while failure is undisclosed, so that even accurate accounts of patient improvements may present a biased view.) Nevertheless, during the 1980s news of fetal tissue treatments for up to twenty different diseases filtered in from Australia, France, Germany, Hungary, India, Italy, Sweden, Great Britain, and Yugoslavia. A respected team of Swedish doctors reported in 1985 and 1987 on fetal transplants in four Parkinson's patients. None of the patients showed lasting gains from the transplantation. The researchers did not give up, but clearly fetal transplants seemed a long way from becoming a miracle cure.

Then, in April 1987, the respected *New England Journal of Medicine* published an astonishing paper by a team of Mexican surgeons.[2] This paper did not discuss fetal tissue transplantation but indirectly raised hopes that fetal tissue could help cure Parkinson's disease. Dr. Ignacio Madrazo and his surgical team described their success in treating two Parkinson's patients by transplanting fragments of the patients' own adrenal gland. The operations involved simultaneous abdominal and brain surgery and were tried on two men, one thirty-five and the other thirty-nine years old, with rapidly progressing Parkinson's disease.

Although the older patient died three months after surgery,

both men experienced immediate reduction of the classic Parkinson's tremors. The article shows pictures of hand movements that progress from pretransplant near random gestures to posttransplant coordinated movements (see Figure 10-1). Ten months after surgery the surviving patient had reached such a level of bodily control that he was considering a return to work. In the same issue of the *New England Journal of Medicine,* Dr. Moore wrote an encouraging editorial titled "Parkinson's Disease: A New Therapy."[3]

Despite the many reasons for caution, this four-page article startled American researchers; this first tentative report of measurable success in the premier American medical journal woke up their competitive drive. As they read the reports and watched the videotapes of these and other Mexican patients shown at several scientific meetings, American scientists worried that they were being left behind by foreign competitors. The report from Mexico was especially insulting to the scientific self-image of the U.S.: Mexico has long been dismissed as scientifically undeveloped, known more for quackery, such as apricot-pit cures for cancer, than research.

Not willing to be left behind, numerous clinics, mostly in the U.S., tried to replicate the operation. Hints of scientific breakthroughs can lead to a kind of gold rush fever in labs and clinics that have labored to solve the same problem. Medical researchers raced to catch up to Madrazo, and by mid-1988, surgeons tried the autografts in as many as 300 patients. In their rush to catch up, surgeons disregarded normal scientific procedures: none of the trials included control groups, none ruled out other reasons for the recovery (the brain surgery alone without the adrenal grafts could have caused the changes[4]), none waited to document long-term gains before repeating this risky double operation.[5]

This surgical gold rush resulted in extreme disappointment similar to that of the recent cold fusion scandal in physics. Cold fusion, or the generation of energy by combining, instead of splitting, atoms, could potentially generate limitless energy. After the press announcement that two scientists in Utah had

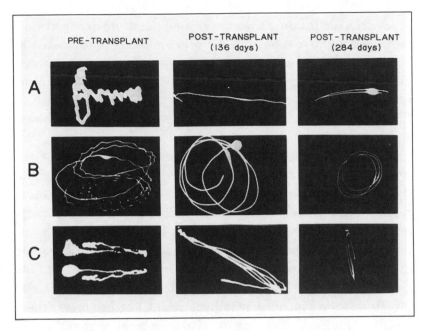

FIG. 10-1. *Spectrophotograms of Movements of the Right Hand Before
and After Autotransplantation in Patient 1*

Reprinted by permission from Ignacio Madrazo, *et al.,* "Open Microsurgical Au-
tograft of Adrenal Medulla to the Right Caudate Nucleus in Two Patients with
Intractable Parkinson's Disease," *New England Journal of Medicine,* Volume 316,
No. 14 (2 April 1987), 832.

produced cold fusion, physicists around the world dropped what they were doing to repeat the experiments. Computer networks buzzed with comments and tentative results, but very quickly doubts and questions dampened and then snuffed out the initial interest. Before long other scientists exposed the Utah cold fusion as a sham resulting from a dangerous mixture of ambition and wishful thinking overriding rigor.

As in the case of cold fusion, failed efforts to repeat the success of the Mexican operation raised serious doubts about the original findings. But unlike the cold fusion incident, these replications involved simultaneous abdominal and brain surgery on very ill patients; autografts cannot be tested in the lab and the risk of severe brain injury from the operation is high, some estimate up to 25 percent.[6] At the March 1988 meeting of the United Parkinson Foundation, skeptics challenged Madrazo.[7] He could not explain why others could not produce similar positive results. Critics suggested that several of the Mexican patients did not have Parkinson's in the first place and that many who had received the transplants were in much poorer condition than reported by the Mexican team. (U.S. doctors examined some of these patients and found that many were in "extremely poor" condition.)

This brief episode of initial hints of a breakthrough cure for Parkinson's disease followed by a rush to repeat the operation and the recognition that the autografts are ineffectual and dangerous, set the stage for an alternative transplant, one using fetal tissue. Although these events should be a cautionary tale imploring scientists to proceed with great care before operating on desperate patients, the autograft episode raised expectations that transplants could cure Parkinson's disease.[8]

As the autograft controversy faded, the *New England Journal of Medicine* published in 1988 a six-paragraph letter from the same team of Mexican surgeons that described marked improvement in two more Parkinson's patients, but this time after fetal tissue grafts. Using fetal tissue, they reason, could prove safer than autografts for most patients since it involves only one operation. In this brief letter, the surgeons describe the donor and the two patients. The doctors removed fragments of the brain and adrenal medulla from a spontaneously aborted thirteen-week-old fetus; the thirty-one-year-old mother had a history of miscarriages and had come to the clinic anticipating another. The brain (*substantia nigra*) tissue was transplanted into a fifty-year-old man who had suffered from Parkinson's disease for nine years, and the adrenal tissue was transplanted into a thirty-five-year-old woman who first showed Parkinson's symptoms five years earlier. After two months, neither patient suffered complications from the surgery and both showed measurable reductions in Parkinson's symptoms. The letter ends with appropriate scientific caution by noting that only long-term follow-up can prove success.

These and other hints of success were enough proof for a team of British surgeons.[9] In April 1988, British newspapers and tabloids ran headlines announcing fetal brain tissue transplants into two Parkinson's patients. The operations were done by Dr. Edward Hitchcock of the Midland Center for Neurosurgery and Neurology in Smethwick, Birmingham. Before the results of the operations were presented at a scientific meeting or published in a medical journal, the *Sunday Times* (London) announced the results in the tabloidlike tales "My Story, by a Brain Transplant Wife" and "I Watched Mother Come Out of Hell." the *Sunday Mercury* (Birmingham) interviewed the parents of a child who died of encephalitis for their story "New Life Plan by Brain Op. Woman." The grieving parents told the reporter that fetal tissue transplants would have given them hope, though no medical scientist was suggesting that fetal tissue could cure encephalitis.

The medical establishment retaliated with calls for caution in the *Lancet* and the *British Medical Journal*. Editorials in both journals insisted that the mere ability to do an operation was not adequate justification for brain surgery. They called for a halt to further operations until follow-up indicated that immediate gains proved long lasting. They also questioned the validity of the reports of immediate improvement. It seems medically unlikely that the transplanted fetal tissue could instantaneously replace the brain function of the advanced Parkinson's patient, but that is just what doctors and patients were claiming. For example, one patient was awake during the fetal tissue transplant—it was performed under local anesthesia—and described the experience to a journalist:

> There I was strapped in a chair with half my head drilled open and surrounded by doctors. Then I suddenly realized I could move my arm for the first time in ages. . . . Millions of cells were implanted in just a few seconds. And as they went in I immediately felt relief.[10]

Despite skepticism that these headline-grabbing miracle cures were really the result of the fetal tissue transplants—it is more likely that such immediate gains are the result of cutting into the brain—Dr. Hitchcock and his team of surgeons repeated the operation three days after the *Lancet* called for the moratorium. They replied to their critics by writing the *Lancet* that "most scientists would not accept that no more operations should be done merely because the numbers are too small to say whether the procedure is useful or not."[11] Time-consuming follow-up studies and the normal requirement of presentation or publication of findings to skeptical scientific peers must not, in the view of these doctors, restrain the experiments of this promising new cure. The Midland surgical clinic had thousands of patients lining up for fetal tissue transplants, according to the press story "Heartbreak of Brain-op Queue." [12] Dr. Hitchcock told the reporter that he hoped that more hospitals would meet the demand and perform the operation. The race for progress had overtaken fetal tissue transplants.

A year earlier in the U.S., medical scientists had also decided to join the international race to cure Parkinson's disease with human fetal tissue transplants. They recognized, however, that any sustained, large-scale effort would require federal grants. The routine request for NIH funding for a human fetal tissue transplant study opened the last act of the American fetal research controversy.

In 1987, a team of NIH researchers requested funding for a fetal brain tissue transplant experiment with Parkinson's patients, an operation similar to those done the following year in England.[13] The experiments required nerve tissue from aborted fetal corpses, not live fetuses, and were permitted under federal law as long as the procurement of the tissue conformed to the Uniform Anatomical Gifts Act. (To promote organ donation, all fifty states have passed laws that correspond to these national standards.) The scientific review panel suggested funding this fetal tissue transplantation study, and the director of NIH had the legal authority to approve the research. He did not have to check this decision with his politically appointed supervisors, but after twenty years of conflict, anything related to the fetus and abortion was sure to be controversial.

Thus, late in 1987, James Wyngaarden, NIH director, wrote his supervisor Robert Windom, undersecretary of HHS, describing the experimental treatment. Wyngaarden's memo asked for a "maximum review" of this promising research proposal, citing the "potential for publicity and controversy."[14] He noted that though the "research will in no way be a factor in a woman's decision to have an abortion and no federal funds will directly or indirectly support abortion," the transplanting of fetal tissue "may be characterized in the press as an indication that the Department is encouraging abortions." (Actually, it seemed that Wyngaarden was less concerned with the press and publicity than the antiabortion lobby, which included Windom, his boss, among its supporters.)

During the Reagan and Bush administrations the federal government strictly followed the Hyde amendment, named after Representative Henry Hyde, a congressional antiabortion leader, which forbade the federal government from supporting abortion: abortions were no longer performed in military hospitals or paid for by Medicaid, and Planned Parenthood clinics lost all federal support if counselors even mentioned abortion or divulged where a pregnant woman could receive information about abortion: the so-called gag rule. Nonetheless, Wyngaarden asked for approval of the research, stressing NIH's conviction that "on balance . . . the importance of the research outweighed any potential for adverse publicity."

Instead of approving the research, HHS banned it, first temporarily and then indefinitely. Windom was a strong abortion opponent—Right-to-Life groups pressed hard for his appointment—and, on March 22, 1988, he announced a moratorium on the use of federal money to support research on human fetal tissue transplant until yet another advisory committee could address the ethical concerns.

Before the ban, NIH supported only a small amount of fetal tissue transplantation research; they spent $11.2 million, or two-tenths of 1 percent of their budget, on fetal tissue studies. Most of this involved animal research, although in the mid-1980s NIH awarded Dr. Hans Sollinger at the University of Wisconsin a grant to study transplanting fetal pancreas tissue into diabetics. The HHS funding moratorium halted only the use of aborted human fetal tissue, but this stopped research at a crucial and crowning stage of development. The animal work produced considerable basic knowledge, but for medical researchers the payoff comes from human trials; they want to improve medical treatment, not just to learn more about fetal tissue or the mechanics of transplanting fetal rat brain cells.

A neurological surgeon at Emory University, Dr. Roy Bakay, recalled that, "When the ban came we did not have enough basic research on fetal tissue to decide for or against using it on that basis, but because of the ban we went on with [transplanting] alternative tissue [instead]. But now we feel we've gone about as far as we can go in understanding the alternatives without seeing a side-by-side comparison with fetal research."[15] Researchers could not say with any certainty that fetal tissue transplants would offer any medical advantage; all they could say was that there was promise that warranted examination. But such uncertainty could not stand against the obdurate views of

the antiabortionist who could not support research that depended on abortion.

Federal funding bans are a recent and powerful force in public
policy. Many aspects of society, from highways to the arts, depend on federal money. In particular, science depends on federal grant support; federal grants fostered the rapid growth and
proliferation of American science since World War II.[16] By
withholding grants, research that depends on highly trained
technicians and expensive equipment withers. During the fetal
tissue research funding ban, Dr. Eugene Redman, the director
of Yale's Neural Transplant Center, recalled what the ban meant
for his lab: without federal money, the research team worked
as "volunteers" and "one day last month we were down to our
last dime."[17] Most neurosurgeons are unwilling to take the time
to secure private money or to perform the expensive operation
without reimbursement. Judy Rosner, the director of the United
Parkinson Foundation in Chicago, told a *New York Times* reporter, "I don't think the neurologists are in the least bit loath
to try it. The problem is the cost. You're talking $40,000 to
$50,000 for an operation."[18]

Withholding money to control research, instead of an outright
prohibition, allows research opponents to present themselves
as responsible budget cutters, not anti-science. By banning federal funding, Windom and Right-to-Lifers in the White House
could plausibly, if incredulously, claim that they were not opposed to fetal tissue research, just the use of government money
to support research that is linked to abortion. The funding ban
provided political cover.

In this way, the furor at NIH over fetal tissue transplants is
similar to the controversy at the National Endowment of the
Arts over funding Robert Mapplethorpe's photography exhi-
bition. During this controversy, conservatives decried the use
of taxpayer dollars to promote art—in this case homoerotic
photographs—that offends some citizens. In both controversies, government officials can censor without censorship by

withholding grants, and scientists and artists are ridiculed as members of a cultural elite that has lost touch with the average American.

The federal funding ban has another indirect effect: federally funded research is halted but the small amount of privately supported research continues unregulated. Establishing guidelines that are sensitive to ethical concerns yet allow the research to go on is exceedingly difficult; it is a task government leaders prefer to avoid. But without legal guidelines and standards of care, privately funded researchers are constrained only by their personal ethics. Instead of dealing with the substantive questions raised by transplanting aborted fetal tissue, the federal funding ban merely washes the government's hands of involvement in these most difficult dilemmas. The ban was, nonetheless, presented as temporary until the new commission, the Human Fetal Tissue Transplantation Research Panel, could make its recommendations.

11 The Bush Years

Another Commission, Another Failed

Compromise

The Fetal Tissue Panel established in 1988 is the fourth expert panel set up to resolve the controversy surrounding fetal research; HHS established three and Congress established one. The new research raises the same questions provoked by the earlier disputes over fetal research but also introduces novel concerns about the procurement of fetal tissue and the medical benefits of fetal tissue transplants changing the incentives for abortion: life-renewing fetal tissue transplants could transform abortion from the tragic end of a potential life to a positive source of healing.

Since none of the earlier commissions could resolve the controversy, skeptics saw the new panel as a stalling tactic. After twenty years of controversy, many scientists were suspicious of any political effort to resolve the issue. No one can argue with the need for an expert panel to air differences and recommend solutions, even if forming the Fetal Tissue Panel was more a gambit than a serious effort to find a solution.

The skeptics' suspicions were confirmed, when just before the commission began its work, someone in the White House leaked a draft executive order that, if issued, would permanently ban federal funding for fetal transplants. Fifty members of Congress and several hundred antiabortion physicians had written to President Bush urging an outright ban on fetal transplants, no matter the panel's recommendations, and this draft order suggested that the president agreed. Acting HHS secretary Otis Bowen insisted that any decisions would wait until after the panel issued its report, but this leaked draft proved prescient.

The two decades of dispute had hardened views on both sides, and research proponents and foes tried to preempt the review panel's conclusions by stacking its membership. Members of Congress, White House staff, science bureaucrats, Right-to-Life groups, and medical associations all nominated like-minded people to serve on the twenty-one-member board. NIH was charged with assembling the group and did so with political care.

Scientists dominated the panel; after twenty years of controversy, NIH was not ready to yield control over research to those outside the research community. Showing considerable savvy, NIH chose Arlin Adams, a retired federal judge, to chair the panel.[1] He was a Republican and opposed to abortion but was considered reasonable, not absolute, in his views. As a judge, he was accustomed to weighing the evidence and putting aside personal opinion, but his background and shared beliefs gave him legitimacy with abortion foes.

Nine of the twenty-one members were scientists. Dr. Kenneth Ryan, who had represented Harvard several years earlier when scientists had tried to derail state prohibitions of fetal research and had served on the first National Commission, chaired the scientific issues subcommittee. Dr. Bernadine Healy, who later became the first woman director to lead NIH, also served on the panel.

In addition, NIH appointed several prominent bioethicists.

Leroy Walters of the Kennedy Institute of Ethics at Georgetown chaired the ethical and legal issues subcommittee. As antiabortion critics later pointed out, Walters was hardly a neutral observer. He had written an influential article that reviewed the ethical issues in fetal research and concluded that the reliance on abortion did not make such research unethical.[2] James Childress, a University of Virginia religion professor and biomedical ethics textbook author, also served.[3]

Antiabortionists insisted on several key participants: James Bopp, James Burtchaell, and Daniel Robinson. James Bopp is an attorney from Terre Haute, Indiana, and has long been active in the Right-to-Life movement. Father James Burtchaell was a theology professor and provost at Notre Dame and an articulate representative of the Catholic Church's views on ethics and fetal personhood.[4] Daniel Robinson, as chair of the psychology department at the Jesuit Georgetown University, had no special expertise concerning fetal research, but he was an articulate opponent of abortion. The Fetal Tissue Panel also included several attorneys and one citizen representative, Dorothy Height, who had served on the first National Commission. She was president of the National Council of Negro Women.

Even before they started their work, the panel composition aroused concern. Research proponents worried that the three ardent Right-to-Lifers would block any solution that allowed the research. Abortion foes countered that the panel was biased in favor of the research and the scientific point of view. Although including strict antiabortionists would make consensus near impossible, excluding them would make the panel illegitimate from the start. The panel was a miniature political arena, in which representation, not expertise, was central to membership.

Robert Windom, undersecretary of HHS, posed ten questions to the panel. Several of these questions addressed issues that had long churned the fetal research controversy, such as the research-abortion connection and the problem of consent. Other questions focused on the new issues associated with fetal tissue transplants, such as procurement, supply, and profit. Nearly all the fetal tissue that is available for transplant experiments comes from legal abortions that are undertaken for reasons that have nothing to do with research or treatment. A woman decides to have the abortion, and the tissue becomes available to researchers, often without her specific knowledge or consent.

The process of transporting tissue from a hospital or clinic to a research lab also raises ethical alarms, however. Of greatest concern is creating an unseemly tissue market. Even in cases where charges cover only the costs of retrieving, preserving, and delivering the fetal cells, processing fetal remains provides a new revenue source for abortion clinics. Preparing tissue for transplantation is a delicate, if gruesome, procedure. Doctors or lab technicians must carefully dissect—or, since most abortions dismember the fetus, sort through—the fetal remains to isolate the specific brain or other tissue fragments. The tissue must be kept alive, tested for abnormalities, properly stored, and then sent to researchers.

At this time, fetal tissue transplants are so experimental that supply issues are largely hypothetical. However, once fetal transplants prove useful in treating a common disease, such as diabetes, fetal tissue will have considerable market potential. The long lines forming at Dr. Hitchcock's clinic may be a harbinger of the future demand for fetal tissue. Fred Gebart estimated in *Genetic Engineering News,* an industry trade newsletter, that a potential annual $6 billion market for fetal tissue existed in the U.S. alone. One firm, Hana Biologics, projected revenue increases from $2 million to $100 million from 1989 to 1992 from fees charged to hospitals for handling fetal cells and tissue. As long as these fees covered allowable costs, this near 5,000 percent increase could be considered nonprofit revenue. The 1988 federal funding ban blocked these projected sales, and Hana Biologics is now bankrupt. Nonetheless, with the amount of money exchanging hands, fetal tissue transplantation will create a tissue exchange or market that invites abuse.

Federal regulations may not, however, resolve the tissue procurement problems. No matter how carefully crafted and strictly enforced U.S. regulations may be, much fetal tissue will likely be imported from countries, such as Russia and India, which have fewer ethical problems with abortion and are desperate for dollars. The need for tissue imports may become more acute if experiments reveal that successful transplants require more mature and intact tissue from late-term abortions, which are rare in the U.S.

Moreover, even if fetal tissue is donated as a gift and no money changes hands, fetal tissue is different from other donated organs. Someone may choose to donate a kidney to an ailing sibling or an impoverished Third World resident may sell one to an unscrupulous supplier, but this transaction can happen once per donor; we have only one kidney to give. But fetal tissue can be reproduced, raising the specter of medical supply firms enticing poor women into becoming tissue farms.

These are some of the troubling issues that faced the review panel when it held its first three-day public hearing in September 1988. Initially NIH wanted the panel to hold closed sessions — closed hearings are permitted if panel members are defined as "individual consultants"—but it quickly shifted to open hearings when research opponents complained to sympathetic legislators. For the first sessions, the panel invited more than fifty people to express their views on the scientific, legal, and moral issues raised by fetal tissue transplants. Adding to the policy din, all points of view were expressed: medical scientists promised new cures, antiabortion activists voiced their moral outrage, ethicists parsed the dilemmas looking for acceptable rules, law professors explained evolving tissue property rights litigation, patient advocacy groups described the pain of Parkinson's and other diseases. From the start it was clear that the initial meeting would not provide sufficient time to air and debate the differing views and a second and then a third meeting were scheduled.

Prior to their last meeting on December 5, panel members circulated drafts of the report and dissents. The final report included answers to Windom's ten questions, several lengthy dissents (the dissents were longer and had many more footnotes than the majority opinion), a brief review of the scientific literature, and transcripts of the testimony.

Despite the open discussion of differences, the votes on the findings and recommendations closely followed preset positions. The three strongly antiabortion members—Bopp, Burtchaell, and Robinson—wrote the dissenting opinions and the remainder formed a majority that favored federal support for fetal tissue transplants. In the debate that followed the submission of the report to NIH, research supporters claimed that all issues and views were voiced, that the panel followed due process, and an overwhelming majority voted for lifting the ban. The panel voted on their response to each of the ten questions, and the smallest majority was 81 percent: seventeen voted "yes," three "no," and one abstained on the view that a mother's consent was sufficient for donating fetal tissue.

The term "majority" is a democratic icon. The panel's conclusions, however persuasively reasoned, are nonetheless the direct result of the membership selection process, not evidence or argument. If abortion foes in the White House and Congress could have appointed the committee, they could have staged a majority vote against the research, and, just as clearly, if scientists had had a free hand, they could have produced unanimity. When disputes become political, "Who decides?" becomes the key question; all else follows.

For the antiabortion transplant foes, the first of Windom's ten questions was pivotal: "Is an induced abortion of moral relevance to the decision to use human fetal tissue for research?" Eighteen of the twenty-one members agreed with a two-part compromise that states that while abortion is morally relevant, because abortion is legal and the research is important, "the use of such tissue is acceptable public policy." The basic conclusion of the panel majority is distilled in this phrase "acceptable public policy": yes, fetal tissue transplants raise difficult moral and practical dilemmas, but, no, these concerns should not, on balance, preclude the research. The panel majority ended where Wyngaarden and other scientists began: the benefits outweigh the costs.

The panel, like society and government, was irreconcilably divided on the morality of abortion. A few felt that abortion is moral and therefore fetal tissue transplant poses no additional moral consideration. The three dissenters were certain that abortion is wrong and that any use of tissue obtained by abortions added to the immorality. Most took the middle ground that abortion was tragic and undesirable but legal nonetheless. Moreover, the majority could not dismiss the medical potential of transplantation, which they felt was also of moral relevance. "The panel notes that induced abortion creates a set of morally relevant considerations, but notes further that the possibility of relieving suffering and saving life cannot be a matter of moral indifference to those who shape and guide public policy."[5]

The panel majority also recommended that before the federal government encourage fetal tissue transplants, they build a legal and procedural wall to separate the decision to have an abortion from the decision to donate fetal tissue. Throughout the fetal research controversy, from that first 1973 protest led by Catholic high school students, scientists have been trying to isolate their work from the intrusion of abortion politics. To scientists abortion was a divisive moral issue that could, and in their view must, be detached from their research; they see a clear distinction between medical uses of fetuses and fetal tissue and the abortions that made such use possible. Like a well-designed lab experiment that prevents outside contamination, fetal researchers strived persistently to isolate their work from the social upheaval of abortion politics.

This wall of separation was to be built of procedural bricks. The report advises the White House to develop regulations which require that at a minimum the request for donation should follow the abortion decision. Moreover, the panel insisted that fetal tissue must be donated, not bought; that no money or other compensation exchange hands for the fetal tissue. They did, however, acknowledge the need for researchers to reimburse tissue suppliers for the "retrieval, storage, preparation, and transportation of the tissue," leaving the door open for lucrative not-for-profit arrangements. Unless the government became the tissue broker—an option precluded by abortion politics—there could be no transplants if tissue suppliers could not recoup their expenses.

The dissenters—Bopp, Burtchaell, and Robinson—did not believe that an ethical or procedural wall could be built that could separate abortion from fetal tissue transplants. At the very least, a woman planning an abortion may know before her abortion decision of the possible medical benefits of fetal tissue transplants. The dissenters agreed with the National Conference of Catholic Bishops who concluded that it was "difficult to see" how fetal organs and tissue could be routinely used in medicine without "a morally unacceptable collaboration with the abortion industry."[6]

Where the majority foresaw the legal and procedural separation of abortion and tissue donation, the dissenters spoke of "complicity, collaboration, and cooperation in evil." Burtchaell used the analogy of an unethical Florida banker accepting drug money and then using the deposits to help his community with socially responsible loans. In the analogy, the banker rationalizes that rejecting the illegal drug money would not stop the sale of drugs, just as not using fetal tissue will not stop abortion. And, just as in the transplants, transforming the illegal profit into community benefit does not justify accepting the money or the tissue in the first place, according to Burtchaell. (The panel majority rejected this comparison since abortion is legal. Abortion opponents replied that abortion should be illegal.) The dissenters further argued that even if you could separate abortion and fetal transplants in the abstract, you cannot separate them in practice: once its use is shown, the need for tissue will become an incentive for abortion irrespective of the sequence of decisions.

*   *   *

The panel presented its observations and recommendations to NIH, where it received a unanimous endorsement. HHS would, however, have the final say. After the temporary ban was announced but before the panel issued its report, the Senate confirmed Dr. Louis Sullivan as the new HHS secretary. Right-to-Life activists initially opposed Sullivan, an African American physician; they delayed and nearly derailed his appointment, not because he was pro-choice, but because his antiabortion views were not fervent enough for antiabortion leaders. Scientists, however, felt that Sullivan the physician might overrule Sullivan the antiabortion administrator and approve the controversial research.

Shortly thereafter, to the surprise of NIH, Sullivan announced that the temporary ban would become indefinite; the Bush administration had rejected the conclusion that fetal tissue transplants were "acceptable public policy." Later Congressman Henry Waxman pressed HHS on the meaning of "indefinite." He was told that the department would, if presented with new evidence, reconsider its decision, but the ban was permanent until revoked. The draft policy that was leaked before the panel convened became government policy by means of President Bush's executive order. Another reasoned, balanced attempt failed to alter the moral politics of fetal research.

Abortion foes in the Bush administration not only disagreed with the specific recommendations of the panel majority, but they rejected the very basis for forming a compromise; the need to balance ethical risks against scientific gains. They rejected reason in favor of absolutism. Undersecretary James Mason, who had replaced Windom, spoke for HHS: "If just one additional fetus was lost because of the allure of directly benefiting another life by the donation of fetal tissue, our department would still be against federal funding. . . . However few or many more abortions result from this type of research cannot be erased or outweighed by the potential benefit for this research."[7]

Everyone agreed that federal funding for fetal transplant research would not encourage a surge in abortions, but transplant proponents could not say that no one would ever have an abortion to donate tissue or that the good ends served by transplantation would never sway someone to have an abortion. Nineteen of the twenty-one panel members concluded that there was no evidence to suggest that fetal tissue research had any "effect on the reasons for seeking an abortion."[8] Mason did not disagree with the panel's observation of fact, just the process of balancing costs and benefits. To him and other strident antiabortionists "one more abortion," though thousands are done legally each year, was one too many.

Even if fetal tissue transplants did not increase the number of legal abortions, abortion foes feared it could create a lobby for keeping abortion legal. The future demand for tissue could, they worried, add another barrier in their fight to define abortion as illegal murder. HHS secretary Louis Sullivan wrote Senator Ted Kennedy that once fetal tissue transplants become a medical reality they could "create a demand cycle, dependent upon maintaining the legality of induced abortions."[9]

Other supporters of the permanent ban rejected wholesale the legitimacy of the panel. Representative Thomas Bliley (Republican, Virginia) said that since the panel did not take a stand on abortion, then any recommendations about fetal research that depends on abortion were morally invalid. He saw no possible distinction between the two issues. He told his committee colleagues that:

> The NIH was charged with assessing the legal and ethical issues surrounding the use of human fetal tissue. However, instead of seriously considering the ethical implication of the legality of abortion it concluded that since abortion is currently legal, the potential for "significant medical goals" outweighs the "moral relevance that human fetal tissue for research has been obtained from induced abortion." This is akin to a slave owner of the 1850's trying to convince an

abolitionist of the economic benefits to be derived from slavery since, after all, it was legal.[10]

The Bush administration sided with the dissenters. The panel was not Congress or the Supreme Court, where votes count; it was advisory, and the Bush administration rejected the advice. Throughout the fetal research controversy, when opposing groups found themselves at loggerheads—and stalemate ensued whenever the issues became politically charged—they turned to expert commissions to search for a compromise. At first opposing groups, but especially scientists, put their faith in these commissions. Most scientists believed that there had to be an ethical means to go on with this important research; they believed that reason would, must, prevail in the end. But by the time this fourth commission was formed, hope was heavily seasoned with skepticism. Commissions delayed rather than resolved disputes, they provided a gloss of reason over an issue driven by absolutist views, and they offered political cover for antiabortion politicians who did not want to appear anti-science.

When observed in isolation the deliberations of these commissions provide a remarkable forum for difficult issues. During the deliberation of the Fetal Tissue Panel, members expressed and listened to irreconcilable and strongly held views, yet there was none of the hateful confrontations that have come to characterize the street protests for and against abortion. Supporters of pro- and antifetal research views sat at the same table, discussed painful differences, and tried to find areas, however small, of common ground.

The mere discussion of these differences is a remarkable accomplishment. On this one dimension, the panel's work, like those before it, presents an ideal of deliberative democracy; the panel created a science "town meeting," a place where civil, not hurly-burly, democracy could, in theory, prevail. These meetings offer a glimmer of hope that people can confront divisive issues in an open and productive way. The rejection of the panel

report raises doubts, however, that reasoned discussion can resolve moral differences; such differences have little to do with
carefully crafted arguments.

Thus, when looked at as a policy-making body, not just a
forum for discussion, the failure of this and earlier commissions
is unavoidable. Commissions, like the Fetal Tissue Panel, are
powerless. Unlike courts, legislators, and executive agencies,
expert panels cannot make and enforce rules. Persuasion is their
only power, and persuasion depends on the willingness of others
to be persuaded. Judge Adams, the panel chair, lamented, "A
commission requires agreement that is as close to unanimity as
possible, to have any effect at all. Without such critical unity,
the commission members simply voice powerful arguments;
with it, the commission can persuade."[11] Adams understates the
problem, since this panel did achieve near consensus but still
failed to change minds in a White House that merely followed
the momentum of its decisions made before the panel was
formed. Reasoned arguments and ethical guidelines could not
surgically remove controversy once moral politics invaded fetal
research.

For research supporters, the rejection of the panel's recommendations and Bush's permanent ban on funding fetal tissue
transplants were the final straws; they were tired of being reasonable and tried to strip the White House of its authority to
overturn research funding decisions. In 1990 Representative
Henry Waxman introduced the Research Freedom Act, a political move to take politics out of science.[12] The irony of a
politician promoting a bill that would reduce political control
over science policy testifies to the enormous frustration felt by
the profetal research legislators; Waxman was giving up on politics and wanted to return authority for science policy to scientists. Although couched in general terms, Waxman's bill was
written to override Bush's antifetal research executive order.

The Research Freedom Act, if passed, would have greatly
restricted the authority of political appointees to overrule the

funding decisions of scientific panels. The federal government funds medical research by allocating large blocks of money to NIH. NIH then makes some general decisions on priorities—a certain amount for cancer, AIDS, and so on—and convenes panels of scientists to review grant proposals sent from researchers from across the country. Once a proposal is approved by this competitive process called "peer review," the federal dollars flow.

The NIH director reports to the secretary of Health and Human Services, who is a political appointee. Although agency heads are in principle responsible for every decision made in their agency, they rarely intervene in grant funding decisions. By long established tradition, scientists, not politicians, select specific research projects for funding. In the history of NIH, political appointees overruled scientific judgment in only one case, fetal tissue transplants.

The Research Freedom Act said that once a scientific review panel approved research, the president and the secretary of HHS cannot arbitrarily deny funding. To halt the normal scientific funding process, the secretary would have to convene an ethical review board similar to the Fetal Tissue Panel, and this board would have to recommend withholding the funds. If the act had been law before Bush's fetal tissue ban, the Fetal Tissue Panel recommendations would have forced HHS to fund the controversial research. The law would give the now powerless commissions the authority to overrule the president and his cabinet on matters of funding science.

By augmenting its power, the authors of this act realized that the composition of the ethical review board would be crucial to the results. The Research Freedom Act carefully defined the panel membership rules. It would include between fourteen and twenty members with no less than a third, but no more than half, allowed to be "scientists with substantial accomplishments in biomedical or behavioral research." The act specified that the panel would have at least one practicing physician, one attorney, one ethicist, and one theologian.

Although Waxman wrote the bill to take politics out of science, clearly he counted the votes on the review board: it was constituted to give scientists a near majority and to make it extraordinarily difficult for fetal research foes to stop further funding of transplants. Congress was not willing to weaken political control over science policy, however. The act failed, and fetal research appeared hopelessly trapped in abortion politics.

12 The Turning Point

Antiabortionists Guy and Terri Walden

Testify Before Congress on Behalf of Fetal

Tissue Transplant

Ayear later, in April 1991, the fetal research stalemate began to crack, not because of any significant shifts in the political landscape but because of changes in the research itself. During this period, there were no breakthrough cures, but as fetal tissue transplantation became more of a possibility, as it moved step-by-small-step from the lab to the operating room, controversy lost its grip. The relentless, if often imperceptible, pull of progress first weakened and then broke the twenty-year hold of moral politics on fetal research. Ironically, the congressional testimony of an obscure antiabortion minister and his wife most clearly marks this transformation.

First in April 1991 before a House committee and again that year in November before a Senate committee, the Reverend Guy Walden and his wife, Terri, told of their decision to have the first human fetus-to-fetus transplant.[1] Prenatal diagnosis had brought the unwelcome but not unexpected news that their fetus had the genetic disease Hurler's syndrome.[2] Although

Hurler's is so rare that routine screening of parents is imprac-
tical, the Waldens were already painfully familiar with the disease: two of the couple's four children had already died of it.
When their not-yet-born son, Nathan, was diagnosed with Hurler's, the Waldens turned to a surgical procedure that had previously been tried only with monkeys and other lab animals.
The operation involved transplanting tissue from an aborted
fetus into Nathan's abdomen while he was still in the womb.

The Waldens' staunch antiabortion views had placed them in
a painful moral dilemma. Many parents, when presented with
a prenatal diagnosis of Hurler's, choose abortion over the agony
of raising and then losing their child. The Waldens refused this
option, yet to save and enhance the life of their son, they turned
to an unproven operation that depended on abortion.

For the Waldens, however, the issue was not abstract or philosophical but intimate and tangible; they referred to their ar-
duous decision as "our pilgrimage."[3] The Waldens told the
representatives and senators of their family and its struggle to
come to grips with their suffering. Although Guy told the com-
mittees that he supported the regulations rejected by Secretary
Sullivan, his testimony was primarily personal, not political.

Before he began his Senate testimony, Guy passed out pictures of three of his children: Nathan, who was then six months
old, and Jason and Angela, both of whom had died of Hurler's
before they reached their ninth birthdays. This familiar gesture
of sharing family photos personalized the issue, just as the picture of "Baby Boy———" brought home the abortion issues for
the jurors in the trial of Dr. Edelin nearly two decades earlier.
The Waldens' testimony reduced the controversy to the question, "Do we save the child Nathan, or adhere to an absolute
moral prohibition against using aborted tissue?" (See Figure
12-1.)

A single metabolic flaw causes the tragedy of Hurler's.[4] A child
with Hurler's cannot produce an adequate supply of one enzyme, alpha-L-iduroidase, that helps the cells break down sev-

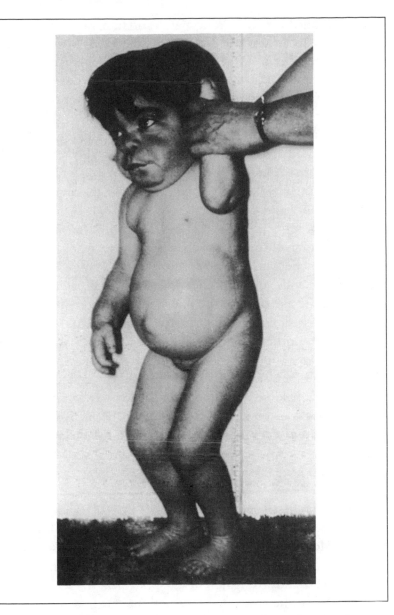

FIG. 12-1. *The Typical Facies of a Patient with Hurler's Syndrome*

Reprinted by permission from D. J. Weatherall, J. G. G. Ledingham, and D. A. Warrell, editors, *Oxford Textbook of Medicine,* Volume 1 (New York: Oxford University Press, 1983).

eral metabolic by-products, dernatan and heparan sulfate. These byproducts accumulate in and distort the cells of every organ, including the brain. Hurler's babies may appear normal until around six months, when a persistent runny nose, repeated respiratory infections, stiff joints, and deformation of the chest hint that something is dreadfully wrong. In the second year, the symptoms become pronounced. Hurler's babies develop large heads, clouded eyes, prominent eyebrows, thick lips, and a broad, flat nose. Hands are often short, stubby, and rigid. The stomach protrudes, and by the third year, the children have heart murmurs and dwarfism.

From eighteen months on, Hurler's children usually become progressively more developmentally delayed. As the child grows, joints become more and more rigid, leading to the contracting of hands, elbows, and knees. Most Hurler's children die before the age of ten from pneumonia or heart failure, after five years of steady regression and eventual total loss of acquired skills. Unlike other disabilities, such as Down's syndrome or cerebral palsy, where parents can see slow but steady gains, Hurler's children start out seemingly bright and normal and then slowly, painfully decline. Except for experimental bone marrow and fetal tissue transplants, there is no treatment for Hurler's, though surgery can relieve some of the physical symptoms.

The Waldens first confronted Hurler's in 1981 while missionaries in Costa Rica.[5] Shortly after their first child, Jason, was born in May 1981, the Waldens moved to San Jose. During Jason's fifteen-month checkup, doctors noticed that his liver was enlarged and his spine curved outward. A local specialist did some additional tests that revealed that Jason had some form of mucopolysaccharidosis, but the diagnosis of Hurler/Schein syndrome waited for more detailed tests made at the University of Alabama Medical Center. There doctors told the Waldens the grim prognosis and warned that they had a one-in-four chance of passing the defective gene to future children. With no treatment available, the Waldens returned to Costa Rica.

After completing language school, Guy, Terri, and Jason moved to the Amazon jungle in Ecuador, where Terri again became pregnant. They quickly returned to Alabama for pre-natal tests, which brought the same tragic news: their baby girl had Hurler's. The doctors advised the Waldens to have a "medically necessary abortion." When they insisted that their religious convictions precluded abortion, the doctors asked Guy to leave the room. They then told Terri that it was her right to decide, but she remained adamantly opposed to abortion. The Waldens gave up their missionary work and returned home to Orlando, Florida. According to Guy, "We were called by doctors from other parts of the country, who we had not met, they called us at home and almost demanded that we abort Angie. We stood our ground."[6] Angela was born in November 1982.

While back in the States, the Waldens searched for doctors and hospitals that could help their son and learned that all medical science can do is treat Hurler's symptoms. Jason endured countless hospitalizations for operations to open up his airways and to restructure his throat. Terri slept night after night in intensive care units and hospital wards, where the Waldens met many other families with children with other birth defects. To the Waldens these families became their new mission.

At considerable cost, Jason and Angela survived. Guy told the senators that the costs were so high that "many times our family caused my employer to have the group health insurance cancelled."[7] But, despite the best medical care the Waldens could find, Hurler's began to exact its toll.

> Our children looked different. . . . And when we would go out into public, people would stare, point and make comments. We had many sad and difficult moments. But they were happy children, full of love. . . . They could not talk well, nor do many things like other children, but we would not have changed anything, if we had it to do all over again.[8]

Although Guy and Terri never wavered in their antiabortion views, they did struggle with the decision about whether or not to have more children. As in all other matters, they turned to the Bible for guidance. The Bible told them "be fruitful and multiply" and did not distinguish between healthy and unhealthy children. Their third child, Hannah, was born in September 1986. The Waldens did not have prenatal screening because of the pressure they had felt from doctors to abort Angela. They did, however, have Hannah tested for Hurler's shortly after birth; she was and is normal.

In early 1987, Jason was deteriorating and the Waldens learned that doctors in Minnesota were experimenting with bone-marrow transplants for treating Hurler's. With their newborn providing a possible tissue match, the Waldens took all their children to Dr. Krivit at the University of Minnesota. Hannah's bone marrow did not match and the family returned home. Before a usable source could be found, Jason's and Angie's conditions had deteriorated beyond the point when treatment was possible. Although nothing could halt Hurler's progression, Dr. Krivit told Guy and Terri that several doctors were experimenting with in utero treatments.

When Terri was pregnant with their fourth child, the Waldens followed Dr. Krivit's advice and had the prenatal screening. Like Hannah, John was spared Hurler's. Then, as Guy told the senators,

> About six weeks after John was born, on January 5, 1989, I went into Jason's room to get him up and he had died in his sleep. It was a tremendous shock for us because he had had a very good year healthwise. We knew that this day was going to come but we did not know when. . . . I believe that it is more difficult to experience the death of a child for a parent, than anything else. . . . Our lives were profoundly impacted by Jason's death. . . . I believe that while we were mourning Jason, we began to mourn for Angie, as well.[9]

A year after Jason died, the Waldens moved to Houston, Texas. Because of his missionary work, Guy was fluent in Spanish, and he became the Spanish pastor of the Sagemont Baptist Church. Guy's Spanish ministry grew rapidly and was combined with a small Anglo congregation at the Broadway Baptist Church. Each Sunday, Guy gave two sets of services, one in English and one in Spanish. A few weeks after moving to Houston, Terri was again pregnant, and tests showed that their fifth child, Nathan, had the genetic flaw.

On September 2, 1990, the police interrupted Guy's Sunday evening service with bad news: the pregnant Terri and the three kids were driving to the service, when Terri noticed that Angie was slumped over in her seat. They drove directly to the hospital, where Angie died, less than two years after her brother. While burying Angie next to Jason in Orlando, Florida, Terri could see Nathan's future: without a medical miracle, he would follow the same painful, tragic path already taken by his two older siblings. The Waldens then recalled Dr. Krivit's hint that researchers were developing experimental cures for Hurler's. They contacted him and he put them in touch with Dr. Nathan Slotnick and Dr. Exmail Zanjani.

Dr. Slotnick is an obstetrician and gynecologist on the staff of the University of California Medical Center at Davis. His practice involves counseling women whose babies are at risk for genetic diseases. Medical science has made major advances in prenatal diagnosis, but for most genetic disorders, Dr. Slotnick can present his patients with only two options: either bring the affected child to term or have an abortion. With rare exception, obstetricians like Dr. Slotnick can offer no treatment or cure for genetic disorders. Postnatal treatment for sickle-cell anemia or Hurler's often involves painful bone-marrow transplants, provided that a matching donor can be found. These postnatal operations are often unsuccessful because during pregnancy the baby has already, as Slotnick told Congress, "suffered the ravages of the disease."[10]

Dr. Zanjani works at the VA Medical Center in Reno, Nevada, where he has completed a wide array of fetal tissue transplantation studies. Most of his research examines the various procedures for fetal tissue transplantation using animals, primarily sheep. Several of these experiments involved transplanting human fetal liver cells into fetal lambs. In one study, the human fetal tissue took hold and grew—what the scientists call "engraphment"—in thirteen of the thirty-three fetal lambs that underwent the operation.[11] The doctors can track the fate of the human donor cells by genetic analysis and biochemical labeling. Only five of the lambs were born alive but all five had human cells in their marrow, whereas three had human genetic material in their blood. The transplanted human cells reproduced and formed tissue colonies that were evident in all five lambs two years after the operation.

Zanjani and Slotnick also worked together with a team of medical researchers on fetus-to-fetus transplants with Rhesus monkeys. In an operation similar to the one planned for Nathan Walden, although for a different disability (congenital hemoglobinopathies), the doctors injected fetal liver stem cells into five monkey fetuses. In four of the five monkeys, the transplanted tissue took hold and persisted for up to two years without any graft-versus-host disease.[12] The fetal transplants became a functional and growing part of the hosts. Prior to the operation on Nathan Walden, however, no one had tried human fetus-to-fetus transplantation.

After Nathan was diagnosed with Hurler's, the Waldens and Slotnick spent considerable time on the telephone discussing the operation. Slotnick even traveled to Houston to meet with Guy and Terri. He told them that the procedure was "very, very experimental." The Waldens explained their opposition to abortion and the moral dilemma they felt in using aborted fetal tissue to help their baby. A few weeks after Slotnick returned from Houston, a young woman was rushed to the emergency room with a life-threatening tubal pregnancy; without an immediate abortion both mother and fetus would likely die. While on the gurney being rolled to the operating room, the woman gave Slotnick her consent to retrieve the tissue for medical research. This tissue was later transplanted into Nathan Walden.

*   *   *

Before choosing the operation, the Waldens turned for help from other pastors and friends, who gave conflicting advice. They, like all parents, worried about the risks to Nathan of such an unproven procedure but also as "Bible-believing Christians" were troubled by the moral questions of transplantation and the use of aborted tissue. As with other decisions, the Waldens asked themselves, "What does God think . . . and does he give clear principles in the Bible?"[13]

The Waldens already knew of the certainty of the suffering and death that Hurler's brings and decided to accept the risks of the novel treatment. They were guided by their faith that whatever the result, it would be God's will. They also knew that, if successful, this operation could bring hope to many families like the ones they had met during their all-night hospital vigils. Furthermore, they believed that successful in utero treatment of genetic disorders could reduce the number of "medically necessary" abortions.

After much reflection, the Waldens concluded that God favored transplants. Genesis told of how God created Eve from Adam's rib. This first transplant, moreover, involved bone marrow and blood, much like the proposed fetus-to-fetus transplant which would consist of blood-producing fetal liver stem cells. Such biblical details convinced the Waldens to proceed. As Guy told the Senate committee, "Not only does God approve of [transplants], he himself performed the first one."[14] The Waldens were also reassured by Zanjani's and Slotnick's motives; they felt that they were "pro-life" in that they had devoted their careers to providing "hope for parents in hopeless situations."[15]

Dr. Slotnick performed the transplant in Nevada on May 23, 1990. The procedure is similar to amniocentesis, but rather than extracting cells it involves injecting live fetal liver cells into the abdomen of the host—in this case, Nathan. The procedure took about thirty minutes. Terri spent the night in the hospital, and the couple returned to Houston the next day. Her pregnancy proceeded without complication until the third trimester, when at the thirty-fifth week she started to have contractions. The following week, they went to Sacramento so that Dr. Slotnick could deliver the baby. Tests showed that Nathan's lungs were too immature to assure viability, but after more contractions and some fluid loss, Dr. Slotnick induced labor. Nathan was born on October 30, 1990, and was immediately placed in the neonatal intensive care unit.

Four days later, at midnight, doctors summoned Guy and Terri to the hospital fearing that Nathan would soon die.

> We stayed until 3:30 a.m. the next morning before he sta-
> bilized. We were really upset, confused and faced with the
> reality that we could lose this child six weeks after we lost
> his older sister. Emotionally we were wrung out. Our hopes
> and dreams were almost gone again.[16]

Dr. Slotnick watched over Nathan in the intensive care unit when Guy and Terri could not be there, and he and Dr. Zanjani stayed close to the family. "They felt everything that we felt," Guy told the senators.[17] After aspirating the lungs eight times, repeated placement on ventilators, and other intensive medical procedures, Nathan came home the week before Christmas.

When on April 15, 1991, the Waldens first testified in Congress, Nathan did not show any gains from the transplant. "I wish I could tell you that his experiment is a success," Dr. Slotnick told the House panel, "I cannot tell you that."[18] At this point the fetal tissue transplant remained just a hope, although for anguished parents like the Waldens hope and possibility, however remote, is an emotional railing that they desperately grasp. "The outcome of [the experimental transplant] may make no difference," Terri testified. "The point I want to make is that we are so thankful to Dr. Slotnick and many other doctors who gave us the opportunity to at least try to help our child."[19]

Two months later, doctors saw the first hints that the transplant might work. In June, they found evidence that the transplanted cells were present and growing in Nathan, but they did not yet produce the missing enzyme. To stave off the inevitable devastation of Hurler's, the Waldens planned to take Nathan to Minnesota in September for a bone-marrow transplant. The day before they left, Dr. Krivit called the Waldens with the results of the latest blood test: Nathan's transplanted cells began to produce just enough of the missing enzyme. The normal range for alpha-L-iduroidase is between 80 and 700 units per deciliter of blood. Any amount less than 80 results in Hurler's disease. Nathan, with the aid of his transplanted cells, was producing 85 units. The Waldens went ahead with their planned trip and additional tests confirmed these hopeful, if minimal, results.

When the Waldens testified for a second time, Guy could tell the senators that, "Nobody really knows how long it is going to take, or how much enzyme [Nathan] will finally have. But he is already farther along than a child who had nothing done. And even if he finally dies, he will be proof that the experiment can work."[20] The promise of fetal tissue transplants was beginning to be fulfilled.

13 The New Political Climate

The Waldens testimony marked a turning point in the fetal research controversy. Not only had medical science progressed to the point where new cures using fetal tissue transplants were imminent, but here in front of a congressional panel was a devout antiabortion minister and his wife—a couple who had personally suffered because of their antiabortion beliefs—asking the senators to lift the fetal transplant funding ban. The Waldens were not just scientists or bioethicists; they spoke as parents of their decision to use aborted tissue, albeit from a medically necessary abortion, with reverence. Their decision was based on prayer and belief, but however based in scripture, the Waldens' decision challenged the absolutist position of many other antiabortionists. Guy told the senators that he too had been opposed to fetal research until he confronted the issue in flesh-and-blood terms. "I would have gone on with the idealist antiabortion position," Walden testified, "but I didn't have that choice. I buried two of my children."[1]

The Waldens remain opposed to abortion; if the elimination of abortion would have precluded Nathan's treatment, they would have embraced that outcome. Nathan's transplant has not, unfortunately, halted the progression of Hurler's. Shortly after their Senate testimony, Nathan's enzyme level dropped below the minimum level. Transplanted cells still live in his body, but they do not produce enough enzyme to stave off the disease. According to his parents, Nathan is doing better than Jason or Angie, but no one can say whether this is the result of the transplant.[2]

But to the Waldens the success of Nathan's transplant—however partial and short-lived—was a miracle, a sign that God approved of fetal tissue transplants.[3] In their view, fetal transplants are "pro-life," for not only do they offer life-enhancing treatment, they may also provide an alternative to abortion for fetuses diagnosed with genetic diseases. In the end, the fetal research issue was no longer black-and-white to the Waldens. They came to view it from the point of view of a doctor trying to help the individual patient, not as an abstract moral principle. "We are the only people who have ever gone down this whole road, and I believe that it is miraculous. I don't believe in abortion, but to let the tissue rot in the grave or be thrown in the trash—we are just letting more children die who might be saved," Walden told the senators.[4]

Another witness who could translate the abstract ethical issues into personal tragedy sat next to the Waldens at the Senate hearing. Anne Udall, the daughter of former senator Morris ("Mo") Udall, told the senators of her father's descent into Parkinsonism; of how "This once six-foot-five man, energetic and vibrant . . . now . . . has extreme difficulty speaking, cannot walk, and day-by-day sits in a wheelchair with his main view being the dome of the United States Capital."[5] She also told the senators how her father had decided to undergo an experimental fetal tissue transplant but his condition had worsened to the point where the operation was no longer feasible. She concluded her testimony by pleading with the senators, several of whom were Mo's friends, to lift the ban, telling them that "This is not an intellectual debate. This is a life and death issue."[6] Anne Udall was followed by Carol Lurie, who had founded the Juvenile Diabetes Foundation after discovering, twenty-five years earlier, that her ten-year-old son had diabetes. She told of her family's struggle and the hope of fetal tissue transplants.

The senators were clearly swayed by these personal stories of tragedy and promise; rather than pursue the usual cross-examinations, the senators merely thanked them, especially the Waldens, for their poignant testimony. Even Ottis Bowen, the secretary of Health and Human Services under Reagan, who approved the first fetal transplant funding ban, urged Congress to lift the ban, saying he regretted his earlier action. "For the past few years I have been out of public life," Bowen stated. "However, I felt compelled to come back into the political sphere to talk about a world where politics should have no place: the world of scientific research."[7]

The testimony of the Waldens and others had such impact because it symbolized in moving, personal stories the power of scientific progress. The steady, if almost imperceptible, advance of medical science eroded the moral opposition to fetal research. Greatest progress was made in the area of research that had received the greatest attention, Parkinson's disease.

At the 1991 meetings of the Society for Neuroscience, doctors reviewed ten years of fetal transplant studies.[8] Although the procedures were not yet standardized and no one was ready to claim a cure, most of the approximately 100 patients worldwide who had received the fetal brain cell transplant experienced some improvement in symptoms.

Dr. Olle Lindvall of Sweden reported on six operations. He injected cells from a single fetus into the brain of two Parkinson's patients, and neither showed much improvement. The other four patients received larger doses: brain tissue from four fetuses was used in each patient. In all six operations, Lindvall transplanted tissue into just one side of the brain so that he could compare the treated and untreated halves. This procedure is similar to giving some patients a placebo in drug trials. The four patients who received the larger doses showed no response at first but after five to seven months were less rigid and could move faster. Two years after surgery the transplanted tissue remained vital, even though dopamine production continued to decline in the untreated side of the brain.

These gradually appearing results and careful follow-ups contrast with the lurid accounts of instantaneous cures and disregard for caution that characterized the British experiments. British surgeon Edward Hitchcock attended these meetings. Even though he had been chastised by the British medical establishment, his questionable research methods had not made him a scientific pariah. Although he had not yet published his results in a scientific journal, Dr. Hitchcock told his fellow neurosurgeons that he had done forty-eight fetal tissue transplants. (This lack of scientific publication should cast doubts on Hitchcock's results, since given the interest in fetal tissue transplants, a top journal would, most assuredly, publish any carefully done study. Animal studies testing these procedures are frequently published.) He reported that approximately a third of his patients did "remarkably well," a quarter experienced some gains, and the remaining showed no improvement.

In the U.S., Dr. Curt Freed at the University of Colorado Medical Center operated on seven Parkinson's patients. To get around the federal funding ban, he used private money, including charging the patients themselves. Four showed marked improvement, and in one case the gains lasted three years. That patient showed steady gains over the first year. Fifteen months after the fetal transplant, the patient stopped improving; though there was no further reduction in Parkinson's symptoms, neither was there any deterioration. Since Parkinson's is a progressive disease, halting the patient's decline is a triumph. Prior to the operation, one sixty-four-year-old Alabama woman could take only a few stumbling steps; ten months after the operation she could walk. "She was falling continuously. Now she can walk almost normally,"[9] Dr. Freed told his colleagues. Network television showed before-and-after videos of this patient heralding that a cure for Parkinson's was near.

These hints of success caught the attention of Parkinson's patients and their families. Although the operation is unproven and expensive—medical insurance rarely pays for experimental treatments—surgeons have no trouble finding volunteers who are desperate for cures, or just for hope. Robert Orth told a reporter of his decision to have a fetal tissue transplant. "I was afraid to talk to anyone because my voice shook. I was afraid to answer the door because I was embarrassed by my appearance. I wanted to be normal. I was desperate."[10] Mr. Orth, then fifty-nine, retired early from his job as a telephone company supervisor in Santa Maria, California. Although not a rich man, Orth traveled to Denver and paid $30,000 for the operation. For him, the most difficult part was not the decision to have the surgery but paying for it. He and his wife, Christine, borrowed money against their retirement savings and asked for gifts from friends and relatives. Robert carved miniature wooden telephones that he glued to clothespins and then sold as message holders for $10 apiece; a task made increasingly difficult because of Parkinsonian tremors. Less than a year after the surgery, his symptoms abated; so much so that he and a friend had started a cross-country road trip.

Fetal transplant proponents felt that requiring patients to pay $30,000 to $50,000 to have such an experimental operation—no one could guarantee success or even define the risks—was unconscionable but the only alternative. For patients, this cost was the most tangible result of the federal funding ban. Most often when patients are included in federally funded medical experiments, the patient's fees are waived or greatly reduced. This is how, for example, novel cancer treatments are tested and provided to patients. Without the federal money, the patients of modest means make a double sacrifice: they take on the risks of unproven treatment—treatment that may, once refined, benefit others more than themselves—and they must impoverish themselves to pay for it.

Although the situation was cruelly unfair, the doctors and patients felt that they had no choice until the federal ban was lifted. As Mrs. Orth stated, "When you are in this position, believe you me, you don't care about the money. You are at the point where you want a little bit more out of life. A lot of people, they will find the money."[11]

Rodney Preston agreed. At forty-two, his early case of Parkinson's was relentlessly progressing to the point where he was soon going to have to stop working at the 3M Pharmaceuticals Company. Higher and higher doses of drugs did not stop his descent into Parkinsonism. "Let [the critics of fetal tissue transplants] walk in my shoes," he told a reporter. "It is impossible for me to relate to you what goes on in even one day of my life with this condition. There is no escape from it. You can't even sleep."[12] He planned to have the surgery in the summer of 1992 at Los Angeles's Good Samaritan Hospital. As one of their first fetal transplant patients, this hospital planned to do the operation for free, but Mr. Preston said that he would have paid if he had to—"I'd sell my house, whatever it takes."[13]

As patients such as Orth and Preston were lining up for this new treatment for Parkinson's, surgeons were already trying fetal transplants with other brain disorders. Ironically Dr. Ignacio Madrazo, the same surgeon who was criticized for the early Parkinson's experiments, was already moving on to other diseases. At the 1991 neurosurgery conference, he told colleagues that he had implanted brain tissue from a fourteen-week-old spontaneously aborted fetus into the brain of a thirty-seven-year-old woman with Huntington's disease. After a year, neurological tests and family accounts suggested some improvement. Though several doctors called for restraint—Dr. John Sladek of the Chicago Medical School denounced Madrazo for even attempting human trials before the operation was fully tested using animals—those who disregard scientific caution and heedlessly try novel operations often set the pace for medical discovery.[14] This relentless transformation from theory to practice also put pressure on Congress to end the fetal transplant funding ban.

Early in 1991, before the Waldens testified, Senator Ted Kennedy had not included a section overturning the fetal tissue transplant ban in the markup of the NIH Reauthorization Bill; he thought it was too controversial and would stall progress on other pressing health needs. Later in 1992, after their moving testimony, the supporters of fetal research found new allies. Republicans Nancy Kassebaum (Kansas), James Jeffords (Vermont), and Strom Thurmond (South Carolina) joined the committee's Democrats and supported an end to the ban.

Thurmond's change of heart was especially telling: he had been a strong antiabortion voice in the Senate, voting consistently with the Right-to-Life faction. Yet for him, like the Waldens and Anne Udall, the issue was personal, not just ideological. Senator Thurmond told his colleagues during the debate that his daughter had diabetes, which might in the future be treated with fetal liver tissue transplants. As an antiabortion senator, he had consistently supported earlier bans on fetal research, but as a father, he could no longer postpone cures because of moral qualms about the connection of fetal transplants and abortion.

Senator Orrin Hatch (Republican, Utah), a longtime leader of the antiabortion members of Congress and the ranking Republican on Kennedy's committee, was not ready to give up, however. He threatened a filibuster of the NIH bill if it ever reached the Senate floor and reminded the senators that all would be for nothing since President Bush would surely veto it if it reached the Oval Office. (The White House had sent to Congress a "senior official" letter promising a veto. The "senior official" refers to the president, but by not naming him, this commonly used ruse allows the president to change his mind.) Nonetheless, the committee voted 13 to 4 to rescind the presidential fetal transplant funding ban.

The 1992 NIH Reauthorization Bill also included a new

woman's health initiative. Women's groups had criticized medical research for slighting their unique health needs, such as
breast cancer, and for excluding women from many studies of
health problems shared with men, such as heart disease. (Many
researchers contend that a woman's hormonal changes during
monthly cycles and over their lifetimes complicate research;
men, the argument goes, are better research subjects because
they are more biologically stable. Women counter that these
differences are precisely why their health needs require further
study.) The 1992 bill earmarked $325 million for breast cancer
research and admonished NIH to include more women in clinical trials and longitudinal studies. The woman's health initiative
was the most innovative part of the bill, but it was hardly mentioned in floor debates. Representative Newt Gingrich (Republican, Georgia) condemned the woman's health initiative as
an affirmative action, or "quota system," for biomedical experiments,[15] but fetal research remained the locus of controversy
over NIH.

The 1992 NIH Reauthorization Bill contained three provisions
that concerned antiabortionists. It overturned the Bush fetal
transplant funding ban, wrote into law the fetal transplant
panel's recommendations, and included the provisions of the
previously defeated Research Freedom Act that would circum-
scribe presidential control over research funding decisions. On
April 2, 1992, the NIH bill passed the Senate with the vetoproof
margin of 87 to 10. The key vote had come several days earlier
when the Senate rejected, 23 to 77, Orrin Hatch's amendment
that merely reworded Bush's ban; it would permit the transplant
experiments but only if they did not use tissue from abortion.

Strom Thurmond not only voted to lift the ban, he rejected
the premise of the antiabortion views in a speech on the Senate
floor: "I do not believe that this bill would, in any way, encourage abortion. I would not support it if this was the case. . . ."
And then, echoing the Waldens' personal story, he spoke of his
own diabetic daughter, "I believe that for the sake of Julie and

those individuals who suffer from diabetes and other serious diseases, we cannot afford to lose this opportunity to develop a cure."[16] Another abortion opponent, Mark Hatfield (Republican, Oregon), was especially moved by Anne Udall's testimony. He changed sides, stating, "I _trongly believe that allowing fetal tissue research is a pro-life position."[17]

During the debate over the 1992 NIH reauthorization, the gruesome images of harvesting babies and Nazi experiments, which had typified earlier debates, were rarely evoked. Opponents no longer directly attacked fetal research but merely raised the more prosaic constitutional concerns about limiting the president's powers and the high costs of the bill. Representative Thomas Bliley (Republican, Virginia) led the floor fight against the bill in the House. In the past he had spoken against fetal research in inflamed, Right-to-Life images; in 1992, he suggested, incredulously, that abortion had little to do with opposition to the bill. After twenty years of linking abortion and fetal research, he told the House that opposition to the NIH reauthorization "wasn't necessarily a referendum on abortion."[18] By the spring and summer of 1992, moral politics was losing its grip on fetal research. The ground had shifted beneath the antiabortion opposition to fetal research.

President Bush, in this election year, also sensed the changed political climate. On May 19, before the House had a chance to vote on the bill, he signed an executive order requiring NIH to establish several "fetal tissue banks" to collect and store tissue from miscarriages and ectopic pregnancies for transplant experiments. Bush wanted to present himself to voters as pro-life and pro-research. Dr. James Mason, undersecretary for Health, told legislators that the federal government could collect usable tissue from 1,500 to 2,000 fetuses a year, a quantity sufficient for all research needs.

No scientist outside government believed these figures; they were based on political wishful thinking, not realistic expectations. One government scientist later anonymously admitted that the Bush administration estimates were greatly exaggerated:

The numbers we used were rounded upward, and upper-limit estimates were always used because we were under a great deal of pressure. . . . What we came up with—1,500 or 2,000 fetuses could be harvested—is literally the absolute maximum if you capture every single specimen throughout the entire country in every circumstance with a SWAT team of highly trained professionals in every bedroom and every single hospital in the United States. No one but the ardent pro-lifer believes those numbers.[19]

Despite the exaggerated figures—Yale's Dr. Redman concluded that Bush's tissue bank would yield less than ten usable fetuses a year—the tissue bank gambit succeeded. On May 28, the House voted 260 to 148 in favor of lifting the transplant ban, 12 votes short of the 272 needed to override the promised veto. (Although it would not have changed the outcome, four supporters of the bill—Pat Schroeder [Democrat, Colorado], Patsy Mink [Democrat, Hawaii], Nancy Pelosi [Democrat, California], and Vic Fazio [Democrat, California]—missed the vote when the roll-call bell failed to ring in the small third-floor room of the Capitol where they were meeting.)

On June 23, Bush vetoed the NIH Reauthorization Bill to, in his words, "prevent taxpayer funds from being used for research that many Americans find morally repugnant and because of its potential for promoting and legitimizing abortion."[20] The next day, the House failed to override Bush's thirtieth veto.

Supporters of the research did not give up, however. On October 2, shortly after the Republican national convention which nominated George Bush for a second term, Senator Kennedy introduced a modified NIH bill that accepted the Bush tissue bank but with a deadline. If, after March 1994, the tissue banks could not adequately supply researchers, then the bill would authorize the use of fetal tissue from voluntary abortions. Even Senator Orrin Hatch began to waver; rather than opposing the compromise, he suggested a two-year wait. Kennedy countered with an eighteen-month offer. After twenty years of moral politics and unwillingness to compromise, the controversy was reduced to bargaining over six months.

The compromise failed, however. Senator Bob Smith (Republican, New Hampshire) rallied conservatives, when, in an unusual gesture, he was joined on the Senate floor by two of the House's most strident fetal research foes, Representatives William Dannemeyer and Robert Dornan, both Republicans from California. Kennedy denounced these "blind extremists" who were thwarting the will of the Senate, but the Senate majority leader, George Mitchell (Democrat, Maine), pulled the bill on the advice of several fetal research supporters. Anticipating that Bill Clinton might defeat Bush in the election that was then just a month away, they did not want to have to wait the eighteen or twenty-four months for the tissue banks to fail, knowing that Clinton had promised to overturn the ban.

Senator Mitchell declared the fight for fetal research over for 1992 as the 102nd Congress adjourned. He vowed, however, that the NIH Reauthorization Bill would be the first bill introduced into the Senate in 1993; it would be numbered "S1."

President Bush lost the election, in part because of his unyielding stand on abortion. His intransigence on fetal tissue transplantation became a symbol of his rigidity. He could not, in the end, be pro-life and pro-science. Although Bush and Clinton rarely mentioned fetal research during their heated campaign, after the election numerous editorials called for the immediate lifting of the ban. The research ban had become a symbol of the intrusion of ideology into policy, and lifting the ban was a gesture heralding the return of reason. On his first day in office, President Clinton signed an executive order ending the fetal transplant funding ban in order to, in his words, "allow more science and less politics in medical research."[21] On that same day, Clinton signed another executive order to free another medical antiabortion hostage: he ordered the Federal Drug Administration to reconsider the Bush ban on importing the French morning-after pill, RU-486.

As promised, Senator Mitchell reintroduced the NIH Re-authorization Bill on the opening day of the new session of Congress. The bill was unanimously approved in committee; even longtime opponents voted for it. Senator Orrin Hatch explained his changed vote: "This is a different political climate."[22] Although Senator Jesse Helms (Republican, North Carolina) spoke out against the bill, even this ardent antiabortionist couched his criticism in terms of government efficiency, not opposition to fetal research.

Except for the spat over presidential power, fetal tissue was no longer controversial. It was eclipsed by a new amendment offered by Senator Don Nickles (Republican, Oklahoma) that would ban HIV-positive immigrants from entering the U.S. After this amendment passed 76 to 23, S1 passed the Senate with only four "nays." After twenty years of controversy and stalemate, only Senators Jesse Helms, Lauch Fairchoth (Republican, North Carolina), Bob Smith, and Malcolm Wallop (Republican, Wyoming) voted against the bill. On March 11, the House of Representatives followed suit, voting 283 to 13 for the bill, and on June 10, 1993, President Clinton signed Public Law 103-43, the first NIH reauthorization since 1988.

In the summer of 1993, the twenty-year fetal research controversy quietly ended as it began in the bowels of the federal bureaucracy where civil servants wrote regulations.[23] NIH was now free to fund fetal transplant studies as long as researchers followed the new guidelines. These guidelines required specific consent from the donating woman for the use of fetal tissue for research. In addition, she must state that she does not know the recipient. Doctors performing the abortion must certify that the woman consented to the abortion before being asked to donate fetal tissue.

The law specifies the punishment of up to ten years in jail for the sale or purchase of fetal tissue or for deliberately getting pregnant to donate tissue, although it is difficult to imagine how prosecutors could prove intent short of a pre-pregnancy contract. The law also requires abortion doctors to disclose any financial or professional interest in the subsequent research. It, nonetheless, allows for payment for transportation, processing, preservation, quality control, and storage of fetal tissue. The ban on payment, moreover, only applies to cross-state transactions, since the Constitution so limits federal regulations.

In January 1994, NIH awarded its first human fetal tissue transplant grant since the lifting of the federal funding ban.[24] The research team will select forty Parkinson's patients from those in treatment at New York's Columbia-Presbyterian Medical Center. To objectively document the extent of their disability, they will be videotaped. In addition, their movements will be measured by computer and their brain activity depicted by positron emission tomography. Dr. Curt Freed, the Colorado surgeon, will then transplant by injection brain tissue from seven- to eight-week-old aborted fetuses into twenty of the forty patients; he will inject the other half with clinically neutral material.[25] Neither the patients nor the doctors evaluating their progress will know who received the transplants or who is in the control group. This procedure should rule out the possible benefit of the operation itself, and demonstrate the therapeutic value of fetal tissue transplants for Parkinsonism. If fetal tissue will provide the promised cures, we will, for better or worse, soon find out.

Epilogue

When, in 1973, fetal research first became controversial, Richard Nixon was president, having just won a landslide reelection carrying forty-nine states, the Watergate scandal was still just a public relations annoyance, and American soldiers were still dying and killing in Vietnam. The *Roe* v. *Wade* Supreme Court ruling had just been announced; abortion rights advocates thought their battle was won, not just beginning. So much has changed in the intervening twenty years.

During this period, prenatal health care progressed rapidly, in part because of fetal research. Rh incompatibility screening and German measles vaccines have nearly eliminated two of the most common causes of birth defects, and surgeons can now repair others before birth. Sonograms, which were not invented in 1973, became as much a part of prenatal care as birth classes. Transplanting fetal tissue may soon provide hope for cures for genetic metabolic disorders, such as Hurler's syndrome, and adult degenerative diseases, such as Parkinson's.

An international team of researchers making up the Human Genome Project are decoding, piece by piece, our genetic secrets so that one day doctors may be able to fix or change faulty genes; in the future, gene splicers may even perform chromosomal plastic surgery. In vitro fertilization has brought the world test-tube babies (though the eggs are actually fertilized in Petri dishes). Several Scottish doctors are experimenting with extracting egg cells from aborted fetuses—a ten-week-old female fetus already has its lifetime supply of eggs—for transplantation into infertile women, creating the biological anomaly of a child having an aborted fetus for a genetic mother.[1, 2]

We eagerly accept many of these advances given to us by science. Expecting parents now look forward to seeing the sonogram with the same excitement that their parents had for the first felt kick. This new technological quickening adds to the wonder of prenatal life, rather than reducing it to a cold, technological experience. But scientific advances are also changing the meaning of the fetus and parenthood; they are forcing difficult and disconcerting adjustments.

The fetus is, and always was, more than just a developmental stage somewhere between an embryo and a baby. It is a symbol of hope and renewal, and its unseen development a source of amazement. Fetal life is the shared story of the human experience: no matter how diverse our postnatal lives, the fetus tells of our biological past and future. Although people disagree vehemently about abortion's morality, abortion, whether for medical or other reasons, is always a tragedy; perhaps less of a tragedy than the birth of a severely disabled or an unwanted child, but a tragedy nonetheless because it forecloses the hope implied in all new life. For parents, the wanted fetus becomes a touchstone for our hopes, just as the unhealthy or unwanted one is a source of anxiety and dread.

Whether a dream or nightmare, the fetus has a powerful hold on us. Except when making precise medical or logical distinctions, most of us think of the fetus as a person. It is not clear, and may never be clear, when during the rapid development from forty-six newly scrambled chromosomes to a baby it metamorphoses in our thoughts from cells to an individual, but this change most assuredly occurs. This shift is part biology and part culture, and people with different beliefs make this shift at different points along the developmental continuum. At some point during pregnancy—perhaps after the first sonogram, perhaps after the decision to continue the pregnancy, perhaps just before birth—the fetus becomes a person in our imagination: we give it a name and nicknames; if because of amniocentesis we know the sex, we may even choose a specific name; pediatricians ask how the baby is doing; we imagine it as a child and adult; we look forward to knowing him or her; we start worrying about paying the bills, finding child care, and all the other burdens of parenthood.

Although not replacing the image of the fetus as a person, science offers an alternative view of fetal life. Science does not diminish the wonder; indeed, the more we know of the complex unfolding of fetal development the more astonishing and enchanted it becomes. Yet to science the fetus is a source of knowledge. Fetal development is a complex biological puzzle that once solved will answer many medical questions. Medical science also sees the fetus as a source of information about the effects of drugs and environmental hazards and as a storehouse of healing tissue. While offering us new insights and life-enhancing treatments, science transforms the image of the fetus from that of a person, or potential person, to that of data and tissue source. This transformation of the fetus from an incipient life to a resource for knowledge or cure, from a subject to an object, is deeply unsettling.[3]

While we embrace the many medical advances brought to us by fetal research, we are troubled by simultaneously treating the fetus as a tissue catalog and as a baby, as a nonconsenting research subject and as a patient, as property and as a person. We want medical progress yet are distressed by the process of discovery that relies on fetuses, especially aborted fetuses, and by the implications of our discoveries. We may soon learn how to implant fetal eggs and clone human embryos, but we don't want to consider the implications of these new techniques; it is too difficult, too painful, and often too far beyond our imaginations.

For the most part, we would prefer to close our eyes to the confusing and disconcerting implications of such scientific advances. Yet, unlike the light in the refrigerator, scientific advance does not turn off when we close the door of our attention. Indeed, when allowed to proceed without public scrutiny science may progress at an even faster pace. Perhaps the greatest danger is not to be found in the scientific progress itself but in our desire to close our eyes to its implications; to, in Langdon Winner's apt phrase, "so willingly sleepwalk through the process of reconstituting the conditions of human existence."[4] This is why controversy, such as the twenty-year fetal research controversy, is so important: controversy slaps us awake and, however fleetingly, forces our attention on the social issues embedded in scientific advances.

Social and political controversy are not without costs, however. At a minimum, controversy slows progress. Because of public controversy the development of fetal life-support systems, fetal blood sampling, and fetal tissue transplants were halted or postponed, and for some individuals, like Senator Morris Udall, a treatment postponed is a treatment denied. We cannot calculate the costs of delaying research on fetal tissue transplants until we see the eventual payoff. If fetal transplants prove a chimera, then few will regret the controversy-induced delays. But if fetal tissue transplants fulfill even a few of their promises, then many will lament that politics slowed science.

In addition to bans and prohibitions, controversy slows progress in subtle ways. Most scientists shun politics; they want to get on with their lab work. Deciding the direction of research is a complex, personal decision, and few researchers knowingly choose topics and methods that will preclude federal funding or will lead to protest or, like the Boston Four, to arrest. Experienced scientists turn to other, less troublesome problems, and young scientists look for other areas of research in which to build a career. Controversy changes the incentives of science and shifts attention away from certain research topics, topics that may yield important discoveries.

Controversy corrodes government as well. Prolonged controversies, such as the twenty-year one over fetal research, foster an ever-narrowing form of special-interest politics. Only the most passionate about the issues, such as ardent antiabortionists, or those with direct personal interests, stay involved as controversy drags on year after year. Somewhere along the way more general public interests are pushed aside: for example, breast cancer research was sacrificed to block fetal research.

Moreover, controversy also creates its own distractions; we look at the fight and the rhetorical blows and fail to see the substantive issues underneath. Once an issue becomes controversial, winning becomes more important than resolving. Difficult scientific and moral questions, such as the ones at the heart of this issue, are reduced to mere ploys and gambits in a political scuffle. Bush's fetal tissue bank was designed not to promote research but to secure votes; it was a cynical hoax.

To the public who pays little attention to the substantive scientific and moral questions, protracted conflicts also tarnish our already dim view of our government; they show it at its indecisive and impotent worst. Commissions, hearings, and floor debates appear as empty gestures, not efforts to define sound policy. To those who are pro-science, allowing antiabortion fanatics to halt research progress represents the most craven accommodation to narrow interests. To research foes, unwillingness to take a firm stand against immoral research, by always looking for some ethical loopholes that allow what should be unallowable, is policy cowardice. No one wins these moral battles over science; everyone, including the governmental referee, has their reputation sullied. People of goodwill on either side are reduced to "Nazi doctors" or "ideologues."

And yet political controversy—protracted, seemingly pointless, often unreasonable—is essential. The social issues implicit in

science rarely receive public attention. Science often proceeds
in small, almost imperceptible steps, with the implications of
the accumulation of its discoveries catching us off guard. Transplanting human fetal tissue followed decades of animal experiments that were duly reported in scientific journals. Except for
the few specialists working in this area, no one paid attention.
Or, as in recent news stories about cloning human embryos,
scientists minimized the importance of the experiment—it was
just one step in the long march of research. The public, in
contrast, was startled by the implications of twins being born
years apart or the possibility of deliberately creating exact duplicates of people.[5]

Controversy creates the context in which we confront difficult
problems. Social and political solutions do not arise from abstract or learned discussion, from seminars or symposiums, but
in the confrontation of difficult choices and dilemmas. We do,
even the staunchest antiabortionist does, want a cure for Hurler's syndrome or Parkinson's disease. We want better neonatal
care and to be able to prevent birth defects. But we are also
rightly outraged by abuses of human subjects, whether in radiation experiments or fetal research, and accept that medical progress cannot be gained at all cost. The fetal research controversy
is real, not just a strategic ploy of politically savvy abortion
opponents.

Moreover, we cannot expect our political institutions to deal
with the changes brought on by the coming biomedical revolution unless we are willing to endure conflict. Any effort to
stifle, or even tame, conflict reinforces the pro-science, pro-
progress status quo. As individuals and as a society we not only
need to learn how to use new technology—how to interpret a
sonogram or to do fetal tissue transplants—but we need to learn
to live with these advances. As a first step, we need to feel that
we have some control over science, that it is not pulling us
toward a future that we didn't anticipate, and, perhaps, don't
want.

Controversy, precisely because it puts up roadblocks to progress, gives us some, if often negative, control over science.

Controversy forces us to slow down, to take a detour. These often rough and meandering detours—detours that may eventually return us to the same highway of progress—expand our language, broaden our frames of reference, and deepen our appreciation for differences and difficulties.

Finding ways for citizens and governments to deal constructively with the life-changing developments of modern science is one of the most vital and exacting challenges of the late twentieth century; it is one of the trenchant struggles of our times. Most citizens and public officials feel too ignorant and incompetent to deal with science and allow, even encourage, experts to dominate decision making about scientific issues. Even though the rituals of voting, hearings, and lawmaking continue, abdicating authority over science to the experts is a central feature of what Benjamin Barber calls "thin democracy."[6]

As a necessary counterbalance to this tendency to let the experts decide, controversy widens the extent of participation. More and different types of people participate, and as they do they learn that while they may not be able to do the experiment or even evaluate the scientific findings, they can understand the social implications of science and meaningfully participate in science policy making. "The taste for participation is whetted by participation," Barber writes, "democracy breeds democracy."[7]

As a starting place, democratic control over science requires that we embrace conflicts, even seemingly interminable and pointless ones. We must, in short, place the value of politics over the promise of science.[8] We can no longer dismiss political intrusion into scientific decisions as a threat to intellectual freedom but must see it as an essential element in strong democracy. Science is no longer struggling for a place in our culture, as it was in Galileo's time. In our time, scientific freedom is a strong, often dominant belief, and we cannot allow scientific authority and the belief that science is the engine of social and economic progress to thwart criticism; we cannot allow research freedom to be used as a rhetorical bludgeon to silence the critics of science.[9]

The "research freedom" provisions of the 1993 NIH reauthorization law represent more our distrust of democracy and our exhaustion from controversy than any real effort to find a constructive, if ever-changing, balance between science and democracy. How do we maintain this delicate balance? We do not have a sensitive social and political thermostat that can keep the temperature of progress even while adjusting to changes in the political climate. Our only thermostat is the crude one of controversy that oscillates wildly between too hot and too cold.

Controversy also begets new forums for raising issues. Protests, expert panels, legislative hearings, headlines, talk shows, Sunday sermons, as well as dinner table and coffee-break conversation, all play an essential role in helping us learn to live with scientific advances. We need to talk these issues out. We may feel comfortable with fetal tissue transplants to cure Parkinson's but what about for cosmetic reasons? (Some European spas offer fetal lamb cell injections to slow aging.) Do we permit transplanting fetal nerves but not fetal eggs? Does a woman's right to bodily autonomy supersede the fetus's need for medical, even surgical, treatment? These, and the many more dilemmas that are wrapped up in this controversy, call out for attention. To the extent that conflicts among interests, ethical frameworks, and institutions catch our attention then at least there is hope that we can understand and learn to live with these scientific advances.

Controversy also changes the role and attitude of the press, which in turn shapes the views of the public. Scientific reporting chronicles, in usually glowing terms, the march of progress. Press stories tell of the wonders of new discoveries and new technology: physicists and naturalists are our explorers, archeologists and anthropologists our historians, and medical researchers our saviors. From the science pages of newspapers to the Discovery Channel, scientific progress is presented to the public in enthusiastic and optimistic terms; science offers understanding, comfort, and health.

Press coverage of controversy changes the tone. Journalists become more skeptical and present the views of critics as well as proponents. They highlight the grisly and the strange, such as experiments with fetal heads or aborted fetuses having genetic children. They seek out commentators who raise troubling doubts and describe the ethical dilemmas. Moreover, controversy has a cumulative effect. Twenty years ago, when science controversies were rare, it took more time and effort by opponents to draw public attention to these issues. Just as in the post-Watergate era the hint of political scandal is almost immediately headline news, now the social implications of new discoveries quickly grab attention. In the late 1960s, fetal experiments that would now be banned were planned, completed, and reported on in the obscurity of labs and scientific journals. With our controversy-heightened sensitivity, the social implications of research often become news before the experiments are completed.

And, for better or for worse, efforts to stifle or channel conflict over science are doomed to failure. Controversy is inexorable and will find a way to escape all efforts to contain or constrain it. The fetal research dispute, or at least the current phase of it, ended in the summer of 1993 with the passage of Public Law 103-43. This law established the ethical standards suggested by the various national commissions, but it also limits the president's authority to block research. The twenty-year fetal research controversy lifted the lid on some of the social concerns embedded in biomedical research; the "research freedom" provision of the law tries to nail that lid shut.

But this and other controversies over science reflect an underlying truth about contemporary American government: citizens and those who purport to speak on their behalf can and will intervene in any aspect of policy that they wish, even in those areas such as biomedical research and biomedical ethics that experts regard as their bailiwick. Controversy, and the everpresent threat of controversy, make policy making more disorderly and less rational; demagoguery is often more persuasive than reason. But controversy, with all its loose ends, inflated rhetoric, unpredictability, and plain stupidity, forces us to confront difficult issues. So, too, scientific and medical progress are enriched by debates about research ethics and by our overall democratic involvement.

It is essential, however, not to overstate the power of controversy and the anti-science, anti-progress sentiment expressed during controversies. At no point during this prolonged dispute did opponents of fetal research, even though they had considerable political clout during the Reagan and Bush administrations, represent any more than a fringe or minority view. With the increase in public protest over science over the past twenty years, the public still supports science and technology; to the public, they are still seen as leading to the good life.[10] Controversy raises questions but cannot assure that we will look for, much less find, answers.

The fetal research controversy, like others in the new life sciences (the Human Genome Project, cloning embryos), raises troubling questions about the human condition, about what it means to be a person. Over the centuries we have developed cultures and beliefs around the unavoidable tragedies and pain of human life: we grow old and often endure debilitating diseases, children are born with disabilities, couples cannot bear children; we endure accidents, indifference, and suffering. As individuals we may want to avoid and, if stricken, to lift the effects of fate, but what will this mean for humanity? Medical science strives for a future where everyone is born healthy and normal, lives a full life span, and expires painlessly like a spent lithium battery. But this health utopia may not be a better place than our current world of uncertainty, disease, and disability.

The dream of medical progress is deeply ironic: it spurs scientists to create life-enhancing cures, but if the dream is ever fully realized it may create a bleak world devoid of difference and anguish. But where can you draw the line between life-enhancing and life-diminishing progress? Should we have stopped with antibiotics, amniocentesis, or sonograms? Should we draw the line at fetal surgery, fetal tissue transplants, or embryo cloning? We have created a science-driven society, and, until we can collectively say "no" to the next small step, what is possible will be realized, and progress, and our devotion to it, will, in the end, trump all other values.

Notes

INTRODUCTION

1. FR Doc. 93-2974.
2. Kolata, Gina, "Patients Paying to Be Subjects in Brain Study," *New York Times* (24 May 1992), A1, A11.
3. LaFollette, Marcel C., *Making Science Our Own: Public Images of Science* (Chicago: University of Chicago Press, 1990), 6.
4. For case studies of controversies over science see: Engelhardt, Tristram H., Jr., and Authur L. Caplan, editors, *Scientific Controversies: Case Studies in the Resolution and Closure of Disputes in Science and Technology* (New York: Cambridge University Press, 1987), and Nelkin, Dorothy, *Controversy: The Politics of Technical Decisions,* Third Edition (Newbury Park, CA: Sage Publications, 1992).
5. For example, see Baltimore, David, "Limiting Science: A Biologist's Perspective," *Daedalus* 107, no. 2 (Spring 1978), 35–45.
6. Proctor, Robert N., *Value-Free Science?: Purity and Power in Modern Knowledge* (Cambridge, MA: Harvard University Press, 1991), 4.

7. Hans, Jonas, "Freedom of Scientific Inquiry and the Public Interest," in *Regulation of Scientific Inquiry: Societal Concerns with Research*, edited by Keith M. Wulff, 33–40 (Boulder, CO: Westview Press, 1979). Jonas rejects the moral immunity of discovery.

8. Proctor, *Value-Free Science*, 269.

9. *Ibid.*, 4.

10. Ezrahi, Yaron, *The Descent of Icarus: Science and the Transformation of Contemporary Democracy* (Cambridge, MA: Harvard University Press, 1990), Chapter 1.

11. Quoted in Piel, Gerard, "Scientific Research: Determining the Limits," in *Regulation of Scientific Inquiry: Societal Concerns with Research*, edited by Keith M. Wulff, 41–46 (Boulder, CO: Westview Press, 1979).

12. Price, Don K., "Endless Frontier or Bureaucratic Morass," *Daedalus* 107, no. 2 (Spring 1978), 75.

13. For example, see Ezrahi, *The Descent of Icarus*, and Proctor, *Value-Free Science*.

14. Fiorian, Morris, "The Decline of Collective Responsibility," *Daedalus* 109 (Summer 1980), 44.

15. Proctor, *Value-Free Science*, 271.

16. Goodell, Rae, "The Role of the Mass Media in Scientific Controversy," in *Scientific Controversies: Case Studies in the Resolution and Closure of Disputes in Science and Technology*, edited by Tristram H. Engelhardt, Jr., and Arthur L. Caplan (New York: Cambridge University Press, 1987), 590.

17. Bronowski, Jacob, *Science and Human Values*, Second Edition (New York: Harper & Row, 1965), 6.

CHAPTER 1: FROM THE LABORATORY TO THE STREETS

1. This medical tragedy was brought into the living rooms of Americans by the photographs in *Life* 53, no. 6 (10 August 1962), 24–36.

2. Later, when her suspicions proved correct, she was given a distinguished public service award for her stubbornness.

3. In the early 1960s, drug companies commonly supplied doctors with new, as yet unproven drugs. The physicians were permitted by law to give the trial drugs to patients without informing them of their unproven status. Doctors would then report back to the drug companies about the safety and effectiveness of the new product. Drug company applications for FDA approval of new

medicines were often based on such field tests. The American company applying for the license for thalidomide enlisted 1,200 doctors for such trials.

4. PL 87-781, 76 STAT 780 (10 October 1962).
5. The increase in the reported frequency of abortion may have been largely due to the change of attitudes and the increase in hospital abortions rather than in a significant increase in the actual frequency; surreptitious abortions were rarely reported and counted.
6. Quoted in Scarf, Maggie, "The Fetus as Guinea Pig," *New York Times Magazine* (19 October 1975), 92.
7. Conniff, James C. G., "The World of the Unborn," *New York Times Magazine* (8 January 1967), 41.
8. *Ibid.*, 100.
9. Quoted in Brody, Jane E., and Edward B. Fiske, "Ethics Debate Set Off by Life Science Gains," *New York Times* (28 March 1971), 54.
10. Quoted in *ibid.*, 54.
11. Peel, Sir John, chairman, *Report of the Advisory Group on the Use of Fetuses and Fetal Material for Research* (London: H. M. Stationery Office, SBN 11 3204787, 1972).
12. Quoted in Cohen, Victor, "Live Fetus Research Debated," *Washington Post* (10 April 1973), A9.
13. The director of NIH reports to the secretary of HEW. The Carter administration created separate Departments of Education and Health and Human Services.
14. Condit, Celeste M., *Decoding Abortion Rhetoric: Communicating Social Change* (Urbana: University of Illinois Press, 1990), 1.
15. Through most of the nineteenth century, however, abortion was considered medically acceptable. For a history, see Mohr, James C., *Abortion in America: The Origins and Evolution of National Policy, 1800–1900* (New York: Oxford University Press, 1978).
16. Eastman, Nicholson J., *Williams Obstetrics,* Tenth Edition (New York: Appleton-Century-Crofts, Inc., 1950), 1043.
17. Condit, *Decoding Abortion,* 22.
18. Two related decisions were announced that day. The *Doe* v. *Bolton* case also defined a woman's rights in regard to abortion but has not had the same legal impact nor public visibility as *Roe* v. *Wade.*
19. Condit, *Decoding Abortion,* 22.
20. Hershey, Marjorie R., "Direct Action and the Abortion Issue:

The Political Participation of Single-Issue Groups," in *Interest Group Politics,* Second Edition, edited by Alan Cigler and Burdett Loomis (Washington, DC: CQ Press, 1986), 27–45.

21. Gold, Rachel B., and Dorothy Lehrman, "Fetal Research Under Fire: The Influence of Abortion Politics," *Family Planning Perspectives* 21 (January/February 1989), 6–11.

22. Cohen, "Life-Fetus Research Debated," *Washington Post* (10 April 1973), A1, A9.

23. Jones, James H., *Bad Blood: The Tuskegee Syphilis Experiment,* New and Revised Edition (New York: The Free Press, 1993).

24. Quoted in *ibid.,* p. 14; original reference, *Atlanta Constitution* (27 July, 1972), 4A.

25. Cohen, Victor, "NIH Vows Not to Fund Fetus Work," *Washington Post* (13 April 1973), A1, A8.

26. Fletcher, John C., and Joseph D. Schulman, "Fetal Research: The State of the Question," *Hastings Center Report* 15, no. 2 (April 1985), 6.

27. Quoted in Cohen, "NIH Vows," A8.

28. Both quotes from *ibid.,* A1.

CHAPTER 2: LEARNING ABOUT THE FETUS

1. Dunston, G. R., editor, *The Human Embryo: Aristotle and the Arabic and European Traditions* (Exeter, England: University of Exeter Press, 1990), 4.

2. Meyer, Arthur W., *The Rise of Embryology* (Stanford: Stanford University Press, 1939), 39.

3. Seller, Mary J. "Short Communication: Some Fallacies in Embryology Through the Ages," in *The Human Embryo: Aristotle and the Arabic and European Traditions,* edited by G. R. Dunston, 222–227 (Exeter, England: University of Exeter Press, 1990), 225.

4. Quoted in Meyer, *The Rise of Embryology,* 38.

5. Quoted in *ibid.,* 139.

6. Seller, "Short Communication," 227.

7. Meyer, *The Rise of Embryology,* 39.

8. Seller, "Short Communication," 226.

9. *Ibid.*

10. Hellegers, Andre E., "Fetal Research," in *Encyclopedia of Bioethics,* Volume 2, edited by Warren T. Reich, (New York: The Free Press, 1978), 489.

11. The dynamics of fetal circulation do undergo pronounced changes as the umbilical vessels constrict after birth; Cunningham, F. Gary, Paul C. MacDonald, and Norman F. Grant, *Williams Obstetrics, Eighteenth Edition* (New York: Appleton-Lange, 1989), 99–101.

12. Hagelin, Ove, *The Byrth of Mankynde Otherwyse Named the Womans Booke: Embryology, Obstetrics, Gynaecology Through Four Centuries, An Illustrated and Annotated Catalogue of Rare Books in the Library of the Swedish Society of Medicine* (Stockholm: Svenska Läkaresällskapet, 1990), 129.

13. Parr, Bartholomew, *The London Medical Dictionary: Including, Under Distinct Heads, Every Branch of Medicine, Viz. Anatomy, Physiology, and Pathology, the Practice of Physic and Surgery, Therapeutics, and Material Medica; with Whatever Related to Medicine in Natural Philosophy, Chemistry, and Natural History* (Philadelphia: Mitchell, Ames, and White, 1819), 674.

14. Agassiz, Louis, *Twelve Lectures on Comparative Embryology* (Boston: Redding and Co., 1849).

15. Lehrman, Dorothy, *Summary: Fetal Research and Fetal Tissue Research* (Washington, DC: Association of American Medical Colleges, 1988), v.

16. Prior to their deliberations in 1974 on fetal research, the National Commission for the Protection of Human Subjects of Biomedical and Behavioral Research funded a thorough literature review on the nature, extent, and purpose of fetal research. This review organized more than 3,000 reported projects into four of these six categories, and recent developments added two more: fetal surgery and fetal tissue transplantation research. The National Commission for the Protection of Human Subjects of Biomedical and Behavioral Research, "Report and Recommendations," *Federal Register* 40 (8 August 1975), 33532–33534; see also Lehrman, "Summary."

17. Cunningham *et al.*, *Obstetric*, 103.

18. For a review see Smotherman, William P., and Scott R. Robinson, editors, *Behavior of the Fetus* (Caldwell, NY: The Telford Press, 1988).

19. Fletcher, John C., and Mark I. Evans, "Maternal Bonding in Early Fetal Ultrasound Examinations," *New England Journal of Medicine* 308, no. 7 (17 February 1983), 392–393.

20. Kolata, Gina, "Miniature Scope Gives the Earliest Pictures of a Developing Embryo," *New York Times* (6 July 1993), B6.

21. "Needle Surgery Saved a Fetus, Doctor Says," *New York Times* (17 February 1994), A12.

22. For a review of prenatal diagnostic procedures see Nightingale, Elena O., and Melissa Goldman, *Before Birth: Prenatal Testing for Genetic Disease* (Cambridge, MA: Harvard University Press, 1990).

23. *Ibid.*, 30–31.

24. The risk of damage to or loss of the fetus from amniocentesis is slight; in some studies, it is not statistically meaningful. This, of course, was not known when the procedures were being developed. Moreover, doctors have learned from experience how to minimize the risk by using sonograms to guide the needle and by the use of narrow-gauge needles.

25. Chromosonal analysis involves examination of the overall chromosomes for structural defects like the extra twenty-first chromosome that causes Down's syndrome. DNA analysis involves study of the specific genes.

26. Kolata, Gina, "Genetic Defects Detected in Embryos Just Days Old," *New York Times* (24 September 1992), A1, A12.

27. *Ibid.*, A12.

28. *Ibid.*

29. Hansen, John T., and John R. Sladek, "Fetal Research," *Science* 246 (1989), 777.

30. Griener, Glenn, "Introduction," in *Biomedical Ethics and Fetal Therapy,* edited by Carl Nimrod and Glenn Griener, 1–4 (Waterloo, Canada: Wilfrid Laurier University Press, 1988), 2.

31. Starr, Paul, *The Social Transformation of American Medicine* (New York: Basic Books, 1982), 346–347.

32. For example, see Gold, Rachel B., and Dorothy Lehrman, "Fetal Research Under Fire: The Influence of Abortion Politics," *Family Planning Journal* 21 (January/February 1989), 6–11.

33. McCullagh, Peter, *The Foetus as Transplant Donor: Scientific, Social, and Ethical Perspectives* (New York: John Wiley & Sons, 1987), Chapter 4.

34. Vawter, Dorothy E., Warren Kearney, Karen G. Gervais, Arthur L. Caplan, Daniel Garry, and Carol Tauer, *The Use of Human Fetal Tissue: Scientific, Ethical, and Policy Concerns* (Minneapolis: Center for Biomedical Ethics, University of Minnesota, January 1990), 112.

35. Hansen and Sladek, "Fetal Research," 776.

36. Lehrman, "Summary."
37. Quoted in Culliton, Barbara, "Grave-Robbing: The Charge Against Four from Boston City Hospital," *Science* 186 (1 November 1974), 421.
38. *Medical Tribune* (5 June 1974).
39. See Cunningham *et al., Obstetric,* 2–3.
40. Scarf, Maggie, "The Fetus as Guinea Pig," *New York Times Magazine* (19 October 1975), 92.
41. Quoted in *ibid.*

CHAPTER 3: FETAL TISSUE RESEARCH

1. Lehrman, Dorothy, *Summary: Fetal Research and Fetal Tissue Research* (Washington, DC: Association of American Medical Colleges, 1988), 9.
2. Gold, Rachel B., and Dorothy Lehrman, "Fetal Research Under Fire: The Influence of Abortion Politics," *Family Planning Perspectives* 21 (January/February 1989), 7.
3. Fox, Renee C., and Judith P. Swazey, *Spare Parts: Organ Replacement in American Society* (New York: Oxford University Press, 1992).
4. This two-step procedure is standard in most animal studies but may not be in human operations; McCullagh, Peter, *Brain Dead, Brain Absent, Brain Donors: Human Subjects or Human Objects?* (New York: John Wiley & Sons, 1993), 199.
5. Vawter, Dorothy E., Warren Kearney, Karen G. Gervais, Arthur L. Caplan, Daniel Garry, and Carol Tauer, *The Use of Human Fetal Tissue: Scientific, Ethical, and Policy Concerns* (Minneapolis: Center for Biomedical Ethics, University of Minnesota, January 1990).
6. McCullagh, Peter, *The Foetus as Transplant Donor: Scientific, Social, and Ethical Perspectives* (New York: John Wiley & Sons, 1987), 26.
7. Kolata, Gina, "Transplants of Fetal Tissue Seen Easing a Brain Disease," *New York Times* (7 May 1992), A13.
8. Noted in Hoffer, Barry J., Ann-Charlotte Granholm, James O. Stevens, and Lars Olson, "Catecholamine-Containing Grafts in Parkinsonism: Past and Present," *Clinical Research* 36 (April 1988), 189.
9. Hansen, John T., and John R. Sladek, "Fetal Research," *Science* 246 (1989), 778.

10. For a review of research, see Vawter *et al., Human Fetal Tissue,* 83–134.

11. Madrazo, I. N., *et. al.,* "Transplantation of Fetal Substantia Nigra and Adrenal Medulla to the Caudate Nucleus in Two Patients with Parkinson's Disease," *New England Journal of Medicine* 318, no. 1 (1988), 1.

12. The letter identified a 13-week-old miscarried fetus as the donor. Skeptics note that the *substantia nigra* and adrenal medullary are not sufficiently developed in such a young fetus to locate or transplant. See Freed, C. R., "Letter to the Editor Regarding Transplantation of Fetal Substantia Nigra and Adrenal Medulla to the Caudate Nucleus in Two Patients with Parkinson's Disease," *New England Journal of Medicine* 319, no. 6 (1988).

13. Freed, Curt R., *et al.,* "Survival of Implanted Fetal Dopamine Cells and Neurologic Improvement 12 to 46 Months After Transplantation for Parkinson's Disease," *New England Journal of Medicine* 327, no. 22 (26 November 1992), 1549–1555.

14. Vawter *et al., Human Fetal Tissue,* 83–129.

15. Spencer, Dennis D., *et al.,* "Unilateral Transplantation of Human Fetal Mesencephalic Tissue into the Caudate Nucleus of Patients with Parkinson's Disease," *New England Journal of Medicine* 327, no. 22 (26 November 1992), 1541–1548.

16. Kolata, "Transplants of Fetal Tissue, A13.

17. Kolata, Gina, "Patients Paying to Be Subjects in Brain Study," *New York Times* (24 May 1992), A11.

18. Goldsobel, S. B., *et al.,* "Bone Marrow Transplantation in DiGeorge Syndrome," *Journal of Pediatrics* 111 (1987), 40–44.

19. For a review, see Vawter *et al., Human Fetal Tissue,* 29–31.

20. Stith-Coleman, Irene, *Human Fetal Research and Tissue Transplantation* (Washington, DC: Congressional Research Service, The Library of Congress, 9 July, 1992), 10.

21. Lehrman, *Summary,* 11.

22. Vawter *et al., Human Fetal Tissue,* 65.

23. McCullagh, *Foetus as Transplant Donor,* 26. These comments were made before some of the more recent reports of success with fetal tissue transplants.

24. U.S. Congress, Committee on Energy and Commerce, Subcommittee on Health and the Environment, House of Representatives, 101 Congress, 2nd Session, *Fetal Tissue Transplantation Research,* vol. 101–135 (Washington, DC: GPO, 2 April 1990), 102.

25. Vawter *et al.*, *Human Fetal Tissue*, 90.
26. Kolata, Gina, "More U.S. Curbs Urged in the Use of Fetal Tissue," *New York Times* (19 November 1989), A38.
27. Stith-Coleman, *Human Fetal Research*, 12.

CHAPTER 4: THE SEARCH FOR CRITICAL DEFINITIONS

1. For a discussion, see Gallagher, Janet, "Fetal Personhood and Women's Policy," in *Women, Biology, and Public Policy,* edited by Shapiro, Virginia, 91–116 (Beverly Hills, CA: Sage Publications, 1985), 106.
2. Legal-Medical Studies, *The Edelin Trial* (Boston: Legal-Medical Studies, Inc., 1975), 3.
3. *Ibid.,* 59.
4. Culliton, Barbara, "Edelin Trial: Jury Not Persuaded by Scientists for the Defense," *Science* 187 (7 March 1975), 816.
5. Johnsen, Dawn E., "The Creation of Fetal Rights: Conflicts with Woman's Constitutional Rights of Liberty, Privacy, and Equal Protection," *Yale Law Journal* 95, no. 3 (January 1986), 624–625.
6. Aristotle and his contemporaries took this one step further and argued that the sperm carried the person with the egg providing only food.
7. Bok, Sissela, "Fetal Research and the Value of Life," in *Appendix: Research on the Fetus, National Commission for the Protection of Human Subjects of Biomedical and Behavioral Research* (Washington, DC: U.S. Government Printing Office, 1976), 9.
8. Callahan, Daniel, "How Technology Is Reframing the Abortion Debate," *Hastings Center Report* 16, no. 1 (February 1986), 33–42.
9. Grobstein, Clifford, "A Biological Perspective on the Origin of Human Life and Personhood" (Houston, TX: presented at the American Society of Law and Medicine, March 1982), 8.
10. Gervais, Karen G., *Redefining Death* (New Haven: Yale University Press, 1987), 1.
11. *Black's Law Dictionary: Definitions of the Terms and Phrases of American and English Jurisprudence, Ancient and Modern,* Fourth Edition (St. Paul: West Publishing Co., 1968), s.v. "death."
12. Gervais, *Redefining Death,* 24.
13. Kolata, Gina, "Ethicists Debating a New Definition of Death," *New York Times* (29 April 1992), B7.

14. McCullagh, Peter, *The Foetus as Transplant Donor: Scientific, Social, and Ethical Perspectives* (New York: John Wiley & Sons, 1987), 110.
15. *Ibid.*, 115.
16. For a description, see Hertz, Sue, *Caught in the Crossfire: A Year on Abortion's Front Line* (Englewood Cliffs, NJ: Prentice-Hall, 1992).
17. Vawter, Dorothy E., Warren Kearney, Karen G. Gervais, Arthur L. Caplan, Daniel Garry, and Carol Tauer, *The Use of Human Fetal Tissue: Scientific, Ethical, and Policy Concerns* (Minneapolis: Center for Biomedical Ethics, University of Minnesota, January 1990), 157.
18. Brahams, Janet, "Fetal Spare Parts," *Lancet* (20 February 1988), 424.
19. Johnson, Kirk, "Child Abuse Is Ruled Out in Mother's Use of Cocaine," *New York Times* (18 August 1992), A10.
20. *Congressional Record,* 98th Congress, 1st Session, S26.
21. Hubbard, Ruth, and Elijah Wald, *Exploding the Gene Myth: How Genetic Information Is Produced and Manipulated by Scientists, Physicians, Employers, Insurance Companies, Educators, and Law Enforcers* (Boston: Beacon Press, 1993).
22. Braude, Peter R., and Martin H. Johnson, "The Embryo in Contemporary Medical Science," in *The Human Embryo: Aristotle and the Arabic and European Traditions,* edited by G. R. Dunston, 208–221 (Exeter, England: University of Exeter Press, 1990), 209.
23. *Ibid.*, 219.
24. *Ibid.*, 218–219.
25. The estrogen-plus-progestin contraceptive pill inhibits both ovulation and implantation. This dual effect is the basis for its effectiveness.
26. *Davis* v. *Davis,* 15 Fam. L. Rep. 2097 (1989).
27. Moussa, Mario, and Thomas A. Shannon, "The Search for the New Pineal Gland: Brain Life and Personhood," *Hastings Center Report* 22, no. 2 (May–June 1992), 30–37.
28. Goldering, John M., "The Brain-Life Theory: Towards a Consistent Biological Definition of Humanness," *Journal of Medical Ethics* 11, no. 4 (December 1985), 198–203.
29. Grobstein, "Biological Perspective," 9.
30. *Ibid.*, 8.

31. Vawter *et al., Human Fetal Tissue,* 162.
32. Prichard, Jack A., and Paul C. MacDonald, *Williams Obstetrics,* Sixteenth Edition (New York: Appleton-Century-Crofts, 1980), 588.
33. Cunningham, F. Gary, Paul C. MacDonald, and Norman F. Grant, *Williams Obstetrics,* Eighteenth Edition. (New York: Appleton-Lange, 1989), 746–747.
34. *Ibid.,* 929.
35. Williams, J. Whitridge, *Obstetrics: A Text-book for the Use of Students and Practitioners,* First Edition (New York: D. Appleton and Co., 1903), 130.
36. *Ibid.*
37. Cunningham *et al., Obstetrics,* 90.
38. *Ibid.,* 90–91.
39. Morowitz, Harold J., and James S. Trefil, *The Facts of Life: Science and the Abortion Controversy* (New York: Oxford University Press, 1992).

CHAPTER 5: FETUS AS TISSUE, FETUS AS PERSON
1. Vawter, Dorothy E., Warren Kearney, Karen G. Gervais, Arthur L. Caplan, Daniel Garry, and Carol Tauer, *The Use of Human Fetal Tissue: Scientific, Ethical, and Policy Concerns* (Minneapolis: Center for Biomedical Ethics, University of Minnesota, January 1990), 224.
2. Quoted in *ibid.,* 233.
3. *Ibid.,* 8.
4. Kolata, Gina, "More U.S. Curbs Urged in the Use of Fetal Tissue," *New York Times* (19 November 1989), A38.
5. U.S. Congress, Committee on Energy and Commerce, Subcommittee on Health and the Environment, House of Representatives, 101 Congress, 2nd Session, *Fetal Tissue Transplantation Research,* vol. 101–135 (Washington, DC: Government Printing Office, 2 April 1990), 2.
6. Field, Nancy E., "Evolving Conceptualization of Property: A Proposal to Decommercialize the Value of Fetal Tissue," *Yale Law Journal* 99, no. 1 (1989), 172; Vawter *et al., Human Fetal Tissue,* 243.
7. Field, "Evolving Conceptualization," 172–173.
8. 249 Cal. Rptr. 494 (1988).
9. Persaud, T. V. N., *Early History of Human Anatomy: From Antiq-*

uity to the Beginning of the Modern Era (Springfield, IL: Charles C. Thomas Publisher, 1984), 137.

10. This is one characteristic of many controversies over science. Often scientific arguments, such as the stages of fetal development, contrast with more emotional responses.

11. "Notes and Comments," *New Yorker* 56, no. 25 (10 August 1980), 21–22.

12. Condit, Celeste M., *Decoding Abortion Rhetoric: Communicating Social Change* (Chicago: University of Illinois Press, 1990), 82–87; Petchesky, Rosalind P., "Foetal Images: The Power of Visual Culture in the Politics of Reproduction," in *Reproductive Technologies: Gender, Motherhood, and Medicine,* edited by Michelle Stanworth (Minneapolis: University of Minnesota Press, 1987), 57–80.

13. Losco, Joseph, "Fetal Rights: An Examination of Feminist Viewpoints" (Washington, DC: Annual Meeting of the American Political Science Association, 1991).

14. *Ibid.,* 3.

15. Johnsen, Dawn E., "Fetal Rights," 604.

16. Lewin, Tamar, "When Courts Take Charge of the Unborn," *New York Times* (9 January 1989), A9.

17. For a review, see Irwin, Susan, and Brigette Jordan, "Knowledge, Practice, and Power: Court-ordered Cesarean Sections," *Medical Anthropology Quarterly* 1, no. 3 (September 1988), 319–334.

18. Solomon, Renee I., "Future Fear: Prenatal Duties Imposed by Private Parties," *American Journal of Law and Medicine* 17, no. 4 (1991), 411–434.

19. Terry, Don, "A Child Is Born In Court Case Over Caesarean: Couple Who Resisted Operation Cite Faith," *New York Times* (31 December 1993), A7.

20. *Ibid.,* 413.

21. Robertson, John A., "Rights, Symbolism, and Public Policy in Fetal Tissue Transplants," *Hastings Center Report* 18, no. 6 (December 1988), 9.

22. Vawter *et al., Human Fetal Tissue,* 215–223.

23. For an analysis of blood donorship as a gift see Titmuss, Richard M., *The Gift Relationship: From Human Blood to Social Policy* (New York: Vintage Books, 1971).

24. Hansen, John T., and John R. Sladek, "Fetal Research." *Science* 246 (1989), 775. See also Prichard, Jack A., and Paul C.

MacDonald, *Williams Obstetrics,* Sixteenth Edition (New York: Appleton-Century-Crofts, 1980), 167; Rosenfeld, Albert, "The Patient in the Womb," *Science* 82 #3, no. 1 (January/February 1982); and Harrison, "Unborn: Historical Perspectives of the Fetus as Patient," *The Pharos* 19 (Winter 1982).

CHAPTER 6: FETUS AS PATIENT

1. Cunningham, F. Gary, Paul C. MacDonald, and Norman F. Grant, *Williams Obstetrics,* Eighteenth Edition (New York: Appleton-Lange, 1989), 2.
2. *Ibid.,* p. 4.
3. Speert, Harold, *Obstetrics and Gynecology in America: A History* (Chicago: American College of Obstetrics and Gynecology, 1980).
4. I examined every other edition (first, third, etc.) to mark what changed and what stayed the same. When there was a noticeable difference between subsequent editions, I examined the intervening one to locate the specific year the change occurred.
5. Williams, J. Whitridge, *Obstetrics: A Text-book for the Use of Students and Practitioners* (New York: D. Appleton and Co., 1903), 419.
6. Storer, Horatio R., and Franklin F. Heard, *Criminal Abortion: Its Nature, Its Evidence, and Its Law* (Boston: Little, Brown, and Co., 1868 [reprinted, New York: Arno Press, 1974]), 108.
7. *Ibid.*
8. Cesarean sections did not replace the craniotomy until the mid-1940s.
9. *Ibid.*
10. *Ibid.,* 419.
11. Stander, Henricus J., *Williams Obstetrics: A Textbook for the Use of Students and Practitioners,* Seventh Edition (New York: D. Appleton-Century Co., 1936), 631.
12. Quoted in Leavitt, Judith W., "The Growth of Medical Authority: Technology and Morals in Turn-of-the-Century Obstetrics," *Medical Anthropology Quarterly* 1, no. 3 (September 1987), 239–240.
13. Williams, *Obstetrics,* 418.
14. Hydrocephalus is caused by a buildup of fluid in the ventricles of the brain and leads to an enlarged cranium, making vaginal deliveries nearly impossible. [Eastman, Nicholson J., *Williams Obstetrics,* Tenth Edition (New York: Appleton-Century-Crofts, Inc., 1950), 1126.]

15. Petchesky, Rosalind P., "Foetal Images: The Power of Visual Culture in the Politics of Reproduction," in *Reproductive Technologies: Gender, Motherhood, and Medicine,* edited by Michelle Stanworth, 57–80 (Minneapolis: University of Minnesota Press, 1987), 67.
16. Ruddick, William, "Are Fetuses Becoming Children?", in *Biomedical Ethics and Fetal Therapy,* edited by Carl Nimrod and Glenn Griener, 107–119 (Waterloo, Canada: Wilfrid Laurier University Press, 1988).
17. Keyserlingk, Edward W., "Fetal Surgery: Establishing the Boundaries of the Unborn Child's Right to Prenatal Care," in *Biomedical Ethics and Fetal Therapy,* edited by Carl Nimrod and Glenn Griener (Waterloo, Canada: Wilfrid Laurier University Press, 1988), 82.
18. Lenow, Jeffrey L., "The Fetus as a Patient: Emerging Rights as a Person?", *American Journal of Law and Medicine* 9, no. 1 (1983), 17.
19. Griener, Glenn, "Introduction," in *Biomedical Ethics and Fetal Therapy,* edited by Carl Nimrod and Glenn Griener, 1–4 (Waterloo, Canada: Wilfrid Laurier University Press, 1988), 3.
20. Hahn, Robert A., "Division of Labor: Obstetrician, Women, and Society in Williams Obstetrics, 1903–1985," *Medical Anthropology Quarterly* 1, no. 3 (September 1987), 263. See also Ruddick, William, "Are Fetuses Becoming Children?", in *Biomedical Ethics and Fetal Therapy,* edited by Carl Nimrod and Glenn Griener (Waterloo, Canada: Wilfrid Laurier University Press, 1988), 107.

CHAPTER 7: THE ETHICS OF FETAL RESEARCH AND THE ABORTION CONFLICT

1. Noland, Kathleen, "Genug ist Genug: A Fetus Is Not a Kidney," *Hastings Center Report* 18, no. 6 (December 1988), 16.
2. Fine, Alan, "The Ethics of Fetal Tissue Transplants," *Hastings Center Report* 18, no. 3 (June/July 1988), 5–8.
3. Hellegers, Andre E., "Fetal Research," in *Encyclopedia of Bioethics,* Volume 2, edited by Warren T. Reich (New York: The Free Press, 1978), 490.
4. Annas, George, Leonard Glantz, and Barbara Katz, *Informed Consent to Human Experiments: The Subject's Dilemma* (Cambridge, MA: Ballinger, 1977), 195.

5. Schneider, Keith, "Scientists Are Sharing the Anguish over Nuclear Experiments on People," *New York Times* (2 March 1994), A9.

6. Rothman, David J., *Strangers at the Bedside: A History of How Law and Bioethics Transformed Medical Decision Making* (New York: Basic Books, 1991), 77–78.

7. Rothman, in *Strangers at the Bedside,* argues that German atrocities were dismissed as unique events and therefore irrelevant to the work of U.S. medical researchers. It is also worth noting that the abusive concentration camp experiments did not yield scientific breakthroughs; most were bad science in addition to bad ethics.

8. Rothman, *Strangers at the Bedside,* Chapter 2. The war also promoted big science as researchers and government discovered how federally funded and centrally guided research could make rapid progress.

9. *Ibid.,* 33–34.

10. *Ibid.,* 50.

11. Jonas, Hans, "Philosophical Reflections on Experimenting with Human Subjects," *Daedalus* 98 (1969), 245.

12. The importance of risk considerations in research that involves children is perhaps best captured in the McCormick-Ramsey debate. See McCormick, Richard A., "Experimentation in Children: Sharing in Sociality," *Hastings Center Report* (December 1976), 41–46, and Paul Ramsey, "The Enforcement of Mcrals: Nontherapeutic Research on Children," *Hastings Center Report* (August 1976), 21–30.

13. Dworkin, Gerald, "Consent, Representation, and Proxy Consent," in *Who Speaks for the Child: The Problems of Proxy Consent,* edited by Willard Gaylin and Ruth Macklin, 191–208 (New York: Plenum Press, 1982), 196–197.

14. Quoted in Annas *et al.,* "Informed Consent to Human Experiments," 205.

15. These concepts are generally referred to as "substituted judgment" and "in the best interests of the child." See Capron, Alexander, "The Authority of Others to Decide about Biomedical Interventions with Incompetents," in *Who Speaks for the Child: The Problems of Proxy Consent,* edited by Willard Gaylin and Ruth Macklin, 115–152 (New York: Plenum Press, 1982).

16. Pappenworth, H. M., *Human Guinea Pigs* (London: Routledge and Kegan, 1967); Ramsey, Paul, *The Ethics of Fetal Research* (New

Haven: Yale University Press, 1975); Jonas, "Philosophical Reflections."

17. Thomas, Lewis, *The Fragile Species* (Charles Scribner's Sons: New York, 1992), 7.

18. *New York Times* (13 December 1992), E7.

19. Robertson, John A., "Rights, Symbolism, and Public Policy in Fetal Tissue Transplants," *Hastings Center Report* 18, no. 6 (December 1988), 5.

20. Vawter, Dorothy E., Karen G. Gervais, Warren Kearney, and Arthur L. Caplan, "Fetal Tissue Transplantation and the Problem of Elective Abortion," in *Organ Replacement Therapy: Ethics, Justice, and Commerce,* edited by W. Land and J. B. Dossetor, 492–498 (Berlin: Springer-Verlag, 1991), 493.

21. Garry, Daniel, Arthur L. Caplan, Dorothy E. Vawter, and Warren Kearney, "Are There Really Alternatives to the Use of Fetal Tissue from Elective Abortions in Transplantation Research? *New England Journal of Medicine* 327, no. 22 (26 November 1992), 1592–1595.

22. Vawter *et al., The Use of Human Fetal Tissue,* 137.

23. Jaspers, James M., and Dorothy Nelkin, *The Animal Rights Crusade: The Growth of a Moral Protest* (New York: The Free Press, 1992).

24. Powledge, T. M., "Fetal Experimentation: Trying to Sort Out the Issues," *Hastings Center Report* (April 1975), 8–10.

25. Some physicians estimate that efforts to better capture and preserve fetal tissue could increase the length of an abortion from the current average of three to seven minutes to fifteen to twenty-five minutes," see Kolata, Gina, "More U.S. Curbs Urged in the Use of Fetal Tissue," *New York Times* (19 November 1989), A38.

26. McCullagh, Peter, *The Foetus as Transplant Donor: Scientific, Social, and Ethical Perspectives* (New York: John Wiley & Sons, 1987), 110.

27. Vawter *et al., The Use of Human Fetal Tissue,* 492.

CHAPTER 8: THE FIRST LEGISLATION

1. Quoted in Lehrman, Dorothy, *Summary: Fetal Research and Fetal Tissue Research* (Washington, DC: Association of American Medical Colleges, 1988), 3.

2. *Congressional Record,* 11 September 1973, 29225.

3. *Ibid.,* 29226.
4. *Ibid.,* 29227.
5. *Ibid.,* 29228.
6. Hereafter referred to as the "National Commission."
7. P.L. 93-348.
8. For an account of growing political clout but failure of single-issue antiabortion politics, see McKeegan, Michele, *Abortion Politics: Mutiny in the Ranks of the Right* (New York: The Free Press, 1992).
9. Antiabortion legislators also proposed but failed to pass the Hatch-Eagleton amendment, which would have declared abortion not protected by the Constitution and returned the issue to the states. Since fetal research occurred before *Roe,* this law may have had little effect on fetal research.
10. Rosenblum, Victor G., "Infanticide, Euthanasia, In Vitro Fertilization, and Fetal Experimentation," in *Restoring the Right to Life: The Human Life Amendment,* edited by James Bopp, 193–200 (Provo, UT: Brigham Young University Press, 1984), 199.
11. McKeegan, *Abortion Politics,* 60.
12. For a list of state laws, see Baron, Charles H., "Fetal Research: The Question in the States," *Hastings Center Report* 15, no. 2 (April 1985), 12–13.
13. The events of the passing of the Massachusetts law are taken largely from: Culliton, Barbara, "Fetal Research: The Case History of a Massachusetts Law," *Science* 187 (1975), 237–241, and "Fetal Research (II): The Nature of a Massachusetts Law," *Science* 187 (1975), 411–413.
14. Quoted in Culliton, "Fetal Research," 237.
15. Culliton, "Fetal Research (II)," 411.
16. Department of Health, Education, and Welfare, "Protection of Human Subjects," *Federal Register* 38 (16 November 1973), 31740.
17. *Ibid.*
18. Department of Health, Education, and Welfare, "Protection of Human Subjects," *Federal Register* 39 (23 August 1974), 30648.
19. Department of Health, Education, and Welfare, "Protection of Human Subjects, Fetuses, Pregnant Women, and In Vitro Fertilization," *Federal Register* 40 (8 August 1975), 33526–33544.
20. *Congressional Record,* 20 June 1975, 20033.
21. The EAB did, however, review and approve a number of in vitro fertilization studies.

22. Fetoscopy has proven more risky than first thought. A 1980 review of research found the risk of fetal loss may exceed 10 percent, see Fletcher, John C., and Joseph D. Schulman, "Fetal Research: The State of the Question," *Hastings Center Report* 15, no. 2 (April 1985), 6–12.

CHAPTER 9: THE REAGAN YEARS

1. Approved by the advisory council to the National Institute for Child Health and Development.
2. The three genetic disorders were: Severe Combined Immunity Deficiency Syndrome (SCIDs), Wiskott-Aldrich syndrome, and glycogen-storage disease, type I.
3. President Carter was an avocate of "zero-based budgeting," a policy that allowed programs to expire unless explicitly renewed.
4. This "nondecision" was never discussed in legislative hearing nor announced in the Federal Register. It merely happened.
5. Fletcher, John C., and Joseph D. Schulman, "Fetal Research: The State of the Question," *Hastings Center Report* 15, no. 2 (April 1985), 6–12.
6. *Congressional Record,* 20 September 1982, 8081.
7. *Ibid.*
8. *Ibid.,* 8084.
9. *Ibid.,* 8087.
10. *Congressional Record,* 30 September 1982, 8082.
11. Pl. 99-158, 20 November 1985, section 498.
12. Robertson, John A., "Rights, Symbolism, and Public Policy in Fetal Tissue Transplants," *Hastings Center Report* 18 (December 1988), 8.
13. Snow, Charles P., *The Two Cultures and the Scientific Revolution* (New York, Cambridge University Press, 1959).
14. U.S. Congress, Committee on Energy and Commerce, Subcommittee on Health and Environment, House of Representatives, 101 Congress, 2nd Session, *Fetal Tissue Transplantation Research,* 101–235 (Washington, DC: Government Printing Office, 2 April 1990), 142.
15. *Ibid.,* 177.
16. McCullagh, Peter, *The Foetus as Transplant Donor: Scientific, Social, and Ethical Perspectives* (New York: John Wiley & Sons, 1987), 1.
17. Kolata, Gina, "Ethics and Fetal Research: Government Begins to Move," *New York Times* (31 July 1988), Sec. 4, p. 7.

CHAPTER 10: NEW FETAL TISSUE TRANSPLANT RESEARCH,
OLD POLITICAL CONTROVERSY

1. This was before the collapse of the Soviet Union.
2. Madrazo, Ignacio, *et al.,* "Open Microsurgical Autograft of Adrenal Medulla to the Right Caudate Nucleus in Two Patients with Intractable Parkinson's Disease," *New England Journal of Medicine* 316, no. 14 (2 April 1987), 831–834.
3. Moore, R. Y., "Parkinson's Disease: A New Therapy," *New England Journal of Medicine* 316, no. 14 (2 April 1987), 872–873.
4. Prior to the development of drug treatments, primarily L-dopa, brain surgery for Parkinson's disease was relatively common. The surgery showed initial but diminishing gains and fell from favor because of the risk to the patients.
5. Vawter, Dorothy, *et al., The Use of Human Fetal Tissue: Scientific, Ethical, and Policy Concerns* (Minneapolis: University of Minnesota Center for Biomedical Ethics, January 1990), 106.
6. Marsden, C. D., "Parkinson's Disease as a Pathfinder: An Overview of Neural Transplants," *Parkinson Newsletter* 66 (1988), 4–7.
7. Lewin, R., "Brain Graft Puzzles," *Science* 240 (1988), 390–392.
8. McCullagh, Peter, *Brain Dead, Brain Absent, Brain Donors: Human Subjects or Human Objects?* (New York: John Wiley & Sons, 1993), Chapter 6.
9. These events are described in McCullagh, *Brain Dead, Brain Absent,* 182–187. The British press accounts, although cited separately, are also taken from McCullagh's book.
10. Shrimsley, A., "I've Got a New Brain and a New Life," *News of the World* (13 November 1988).
11. Hitchcock, E. R., C. Clough, R. Hughes, and B. Kenny, "Embryos and Parkinson's Disease," *Lancet* 1 (1988), 1274.
12. "Heartbreak of Brain-op Queue," *Sunday Mercury* (Birmingham, England; 20 November 1988).
13. This intramural grant request came from government researchers in the National Institute of Neurological and Communicate Disorders and Stroke, one of the national institutes.
14. Childress, James F., "Deliberations of the Human Fetal Transplantation Research Panel," in *Biomedical Politics,* edited by Kathi E. Hanna, 215–248 (Washington, DC: National Academy Press, 1991), 216.
15. Clemmitt, Marcia, "Fetal Tissue Research Uncertainties Foster Confusion Among Many Bioscience Workers," *Scientist* (20 July 1992), 6.

16. Smith, Bruce L. R., *American Science Policy Since World War II* (Washington, DC: The Brookings Institution, 1990).
17. *Ibid.*
18. Kolata, Gina, "Transplants of Fetal Tissue Seen Easing a Brain Disease," *New York Times* (7 May 1992), A13.

CHAPTER 11: THE BUSH YEARS

1. Adams was later appointed as an independent counsel examining Reagan era scandals in the Department of Housing and Urban Affairs; see Labaton, Stephen, "Ex-Official Convicted in HUD Scandal," *New York Times* (27 October 1992), A8.
2. Walters, Leroy, "Ethical Issues in Fetal Research: A Look Back and a Look Forward," *Clinical Research* 36, no. 3 (1988), 209–214.
3. Beauchamp, Tom, and James Childress, *Principles of Biomedical Ethics,* Third Edition (New York: Oxford University Press, 1989).
4. Late in 1991, Burtchaell was forced to resign his teaching post amid accusations of sexual misconduct; see "Priest Resigns Post at Notre Dame Amid Accusations of Sex Abuse," *New York Times* (3 December 1991), A20.
5. U.S. Congress, Committee on Energy and Commerce, Subcommittee on Health and the Environment, House of Representatives, 101 Congress, 2nd Session, *Fetal Tissue Transplantation Research,* vol. 101–135, (Washington, DC: General Printing Office, 2 April 1990), 22.
6. Boffey, Philip M., "Using Fetal Tissue as a Cure Debated," *New York Times* (15 September 1988), A31.
7. Secretary Mason, quoted in U.S. Congress, *Fetal Tissue Transplantation,* 17.
8. U.S. Congress, *Fetal Tissue Transplantation,* 24.
9. Letter from Louis Sullivan, HHS Secretary, to Senator Edward Kennedy, February 4, 1992.
10. *Ibid.,* 3.
11. Childress, James F., "Deliberations of the Human Fetal Transplantation Panel," in *Biomedical Politics,* edited by Kathi E. Hanna, 215–248 (Washington, DC: National Academy Press, 1991), 216.
12. U.S. Congress, "Research Freedom Act of 1990," vol. HR 545618 (December 1990).

CHAPTER 12: THE TURNING POINT

1. U.S. Congress, House, Committee on Energy and Commerce, NIH Reauthorization (Washington, DC: U.S. Government Printing Office, April 15 and 16, 1991), and U.S. Congress, Senate, Committee on Labor and Human Resources, *Finding Medical Cures: The Promise of Fetal Tissue Transplantation Research* (Washington, DC: U.S. Government Printing Office, November 21, 1991). The Waldens' testimony was nearly identical on both occasions and will be treated in the discussion as a single source.

2. Hurler's is a rare, inherited condition caused by an enzyme defect, in which, due to a problem in metabolism, there is an abnormal accumulation of substances called mucopolysaccharides in the tissues.

3. U.S. Senate, *Finding Medical Cures,* 23.

4. For a medical description see, Wyngaarden, James B., Lloyd H. Smith, and J. Claude Bennett, editors, *Cecil Textbook of Medicine,* Nineteenth Edition (Philadelphia, W. B. Saunders Co., 1992), 1120–1121.

5. These details are taken from the Walden's Senate testimony; U.S. Senate, *Finding Medical Cures,* 23–29.

6. *Ibid.,* 23.

7. *Ibid.,* 24.

8. *Ibid.*

9. *Ibid.,* 24–25.

10. U.S. House, NIH Reauthorization, 140.

11. Zanjani, E. D., M. G. Pallavicini, J. L. Ascensad, A. W. Flake, R. G. Langlois, M. Reitsma, F. R. Mackintosh, D. Stutes, M. R. Harrison, and M. Tavassoli, "Engraftment and Long-Term Expression of Human Fetal Hemopoietic Stem Cells in Sheep Following Transplantation In Utero," *Journal of Clinical Investigation* 89, no. 4 (1992), 1178–1188.

12. Harrision, M. R., R. N. Slotnick, T. M. Crombleholme, M. S. Golbus, A. F. Tarantal, and E. D. Zanjani, "In-utero Transplantation of Fetal Liver Haemopoietic Stem Cells in Monkeys," *Lancet* 2, no. 8677 (16 December 1989), 1425–1427.

13. U.S. Senate, *Finding Medical Cures,* 25.

14. *Ibid.,* 26.

15. *Ibid.*

16. *Ibid.,* 27.

17. *Ibid.*

18. U.S. House, NIH Reauthorization, 141.
19. *Ibid.,* 128.
20. Quoted in Hilts, Philip J., "Fetus-to-Fetus Transplant Is Said to Block a Deadly Defect," *New York Times* (21 November 1991), A14.

CHAPTER 13: THE NEW POLITICAL CLIMATE
 1. Quoted in Hilts, Philip J., "Fetus-to-Fetus Transplant Is Said to Block a Deadly Defect," *New York Times* (21 November 1991), A14.
 2. Personal interview on February 7, 1994.
 3. Hilts, "Fetus-to-Fetus."
 4. *Ibid.*
 5. U.S. Congress, Senate, Committee on Labor and Human Resources, *Finding Medical Cures: The Promise of Fetal Tissue Transplantation Research* (Washington, DC: U.S. Government Printing Office, 1991), 37.
 6. *Ibid.,* 39.
 7. Hilts, Philip J., "Congress Urged to Lift Ban on Fetal-Tissue Research," *New York Times* (27 May 1992), A7.
 8. Blakeslee, Sandra, "Fetal Cell Transplants Show Early Promise in Parkinson Patients," *New York Times* (12 November 1991), B6.
 9. Kolata, Gina, "Transplants of Fetal Tissue Seen Easing a Brain Disease," *New York Times* (7 May 1992), A13.
10. Kolata, Gina, "Patients Paying to Be Subjects in Brain Study," *New York Times* (24 May 1992), A1.
11. *Ibid.,* A11.
12. *Ibid.*
13. *Ibid.*
14. For a more detailed discussion of this issue see, Rothman, David J., *Strangers at the Bedside: A History of How Law and Bioethics Transformed Medical Decision Making* (New York: Basic Books, 1991).
15. Clymer, Adam, "House Vote Lets Stand Ban on Fetal Tissue Research," *New York Times* (25 June 1992), A19.
16. "Fetal Research," Congressional Quarterly Almanac, 102 Congress, 2nd Session, vol. 48 (Washington, DC: Congressional Quarterly, Inc., 1992), 394.
17. *Ibid.*

18. Hilts, Philip J., "House Backs Fetal Research But Veto by Bush Is Likely," *New York Times* (29 May 1992), A9.
19. Hilts, Philip J., "Fetal-Tissue Bank Not Viable Option, Agency Memo Says," *New York Times* (27 July 1992), A1–A7.
20. Clymer, Adam, "House Vote Lets Stand Ban on Fetal Tissue Research," *New York Times* (25 June 1992), A19.
21. This was how Clinton defended his action in a June press conference, *New York Times* (16 June 1993), A10.
22. Mills, Mike, "With Fetal Tissue Ban Lifted, NIH Bill Has New Problem," *Congressional Quarterly* 41, no. 5 (30 January 1993), 224.
23. *Federal Register* 58, no. 166 (30 August 1993), 45496.
24. "Fetal-Tissue Study Approved, The First Since the Ban Was Lifted," *New York Times* (5 January 1994), A7.
25. Doing brain surgery on control patients who are not expected to benefit has, however, raised ethical concerns; see "New Fight Over Fetal Tissue Grafts," *Science* 263 (4 February 1994), 600–601.

EPILOGUE

1. Kolata, Gina, "Fetal Ovary Transplant Is Envisioned," *New York Times* (6 January 1994).
2. One of our common beliefs is that our genes make us unique, though the genes of different people, even those of different races, are nearly identical. Our own personal genetic code tells more about our shared humanity than our individuality; our genetic parents are more the gene pool than any two individuals.
3. Nelkin, Dorothy, editor, *Controversy: Politics of Technical Decisions,* Third Edition (Newbury Park, CA: Sage Publications, 1992), x.
4. Winner, Langdon, *The Whale and the Reactor: A Search for Limits in an Age of High Technology* (Chicago: University of Chicago Press, 1986), 10.
5. Sawyer, Kathy, "Researchers Clone Human Embryo Cells," *Washington Post* (25 October 1993), A4.
6. Barber, Benjamin R., *Strong Democracy: Participatory Politics for a New Age* (Berkeley: University of California Press, 1984).
7. *Ibid.,* 265.
8. Fielder, John, "Autonomous Technology, Democracy, and the NIMBYs," in *Democracy in a Technological Society,* edited by Lang-

don Winner, 105–121 (Boston: Kluwer Academic Publishers, 1992), 113.

9. For a full discussion of this point, see Proctor, Robert N., *Value-Free Science?: Purity and Power in Modern Knowledge* (Cambridge: Harvard University Press, 1991).

10. Miller, Jon, *The Public Understanding of Science and Technology in the United States, 1990* (Washington, DC: National Science Foundation, December 1990).

Bibliography

BOOKS AND BOOK CHAPTERS

Annas, George, Leonard Glantz, and Barbara Katz. *Informed Consent to Human Experiments: The Subject's Dilemma.* Cambridge, MA: Ballinger, 1977.

Barber, Benjamin R. *Strong Democracy: Participatory Politics for a New Age.* Berkeley, CA: University of California Press, 1984.

Beauchamp, Tom, and James Childress. *Principles of Biomedical Ethics,* Third Edition. New York: Oxford Press, 1989.

Bell, Robert. *Impure Science: Fraud, Compromise, and Political Influence in Scientific Research.* New York: John Wiley & Sons, 1992.

Braude, Peter R., and Martin H. Johnson. "The Embryo in Contemporary Medical Science," in *The Human Embryo: Aristotle and the Arabic and European Tradition,* edited by G. R. Dunston, 208–221. Exeter, England: University of Exeter Press, 1990.

Bronowski, Jacob. *Science and Human Values,* Second Edition. New York: Harper & Row, 1965.

Caplan, Arthur L. *"If I Were a Rich Man Could I Buy a Pancreas?"* and

Other Essays on the Ethics of Health Care. Bloomington, IN: Indiana University Press, 1992.

Childress, James F. "Deliberations of the Human Fetal Transplantation Research Panel," in *Biomedical Politics,* edited by Kathi E. Hanna, 215–248. Washington, DC: National Academy Press, 1991.

Colen, B. D. *Hard Choices: Mixed Blessings of Modern Medical Technology.* New York: G. P. Putnam's Sons, 1986.

Condit, Celeste Michelle. *Decoding Abortion Rhetoric: Communicating Social Change.* Urbana, IL: University of Illinois Press, 1990.

Craig, Barbara H., and David M. O'Brien. *Abortion and American Politics.* Chatham, NJ: Chatham House Publishers, 1992.

Edwards, Robert G. *Life Before Birth: Reflections on the Embryo Debate.* New York: Basic Books, 1989.

Eisenstein, Zillah R. *The Female Body and the Law.* Berkeley, CA: University of California Press, 1988.

Englehardt, H. Tristram, and Arthur L. Caplan, editors. *Scientific Controversies: Case Studies in the Resolution and Closure of Disputes in Science and Technology.* New York: Cambridge University Press, 1987.

Ezrahi, Yaron. *The Descent of Icarus: Science and the Transformation of Contemporary Democracy.* Cambridge, MA: Harvard University Press, 1990.

Faden, Ruth R., and Tom L. Beauchamp. *A History and Theory of Informed Consent.* New York: Oxford University Press, 1986.

Gallagher, Janet. "Fetal Personhood and Women's Policy," in *Women, Biology, and Public Policy,* edited by Virginia Shapiro, 91–116. Beverly Hills, CA: Sage Publications, 1985.

Gaylin, Willard, and Ruth Macklin, editors. *Who Speaks for the Child: The Problems of Proxy Consent.* New York: Plenum Press, 1982.

Gervais, Karen G. *Redefining Death.* New Haven: Yale University Press, 1987.

Grobstein, Clifford. *Science and the Unborn: Choosing Human Futures.* New York: Basic Books, 1988.

Hanna, Kathi E., editor. *Biomedical Politics.* Washington, DC: National Academy Press, 1991.

Hellegers, Andre E. "Fetal Research," in *Encyclopedia of Bioethics,* Volume 2, edited by Warren T. Reich. New York: The Free Press, 1978.

Hertz, Sue. *Caught in the Crossfire: A Year on Abortion's Front Line.* Englewood Cliffs, NJ: Prentice-Hall, 1991.

Jaspers, James M., and Dorothy Nelkin. *The Animal Rights Crusade: The Growth of a Moral Protest.* New York: The Free Press, 1992.

LaFollette, Marcel C. *Making Science Our Own: Public Images of Science.* Chicago: University of Chicago Press, 1990.

Mansbridge, Jane J. *Beyond Adversary Democracy.* New York: Basic Books, Inc., 1980.

McCullagh, Peter. *The Foetus as Transplant Donor: Scientific, Social, and Ethical Perspectives.* New York: John Wiley & Sons, 1987.

McCullagh, Peter. *Brain Dead, Brain Absent, Brain Donors: Human Subjects or Human Objects?* New York: John Wiley & Sons, 1993.

McKeegan, Michele. *Abortion Politics: Mutiny in the Ranks of the Right.* New York: The Free Press, 1992.

Mohr, James C. *Abortion in America: The Origins and Evolution of National Policy, 1800–1900.* New York: Oxford University Press, 1978.

Morowitz, Harold J., and James S. Trefil. *The Facts of Life: Science and the Abortion Controversy.* New York: Oxford University Press, 1992.

Nightingale, Elena O., and Melissa Goldman. *Before Birth: Prenatal Testing for Genetic Disease.* Cambridge, MA: Harvard University Press, 1990.

Oakley, Ann. *The Captured Womb: A History of the Medical Care of Pregnant Women.* New York: Basil Blackwell, 1984.

Petchesky, Rosalind P. "Foetal Images: The Power of Visual Culture in the Politics of Reproduction," in *Reproductive Technologies: Gender, Motherhood, and Medicine,* edited by Michelle Stanworth, 57–80. Minneapolis: University of Minnesota Press, 1987.

Petchesky, Rosalind P. *Abortion and Woman's Choice: The State, Sexuality, and Reproductive Freedom,* Revised Edition. Boston: Northeastern University Press, 1990.

Proctor, Robert N. *Value-free Science?: Purity and Power in Modern Knowledge.* Cambridge, MA: Harvard University Press, 1991.

Ramsey, Paul. *The Patient as Person.* New Haven, CT: Yale University Press, 1970.

Rothman, David J. *Strangers at the Bedside: A History of How Law and Bioethics Transformed Medical Decision Making.* New York: Basic Books, 1991.

Rouse, Joseph. *Knowledge and Power: Toward a Political Philosophy of Science.* Ithaca, NY: Cornell University Press, 1987.

Smith, Bruce L. R. *American Science Policy Since World War II.* Washington, DC: The Brookings Institution, 1990.

Starr, Paul. *The Social Transformation of American Medicine.* New York: Basic Books, 1982.

Steinbock, Bonnie. *Life Before Birth: The Moral and Legal Status of Embryos and Fetuses.* New York: Oxford University Press, 1992.

Thomas, Lewis. *The Fragile Species.* New York: Scribner's, 1992.

Tribe, Lawrence H. *Abortion: The Clash of Absolutes.* New York: W. W. Norton & Company, 1990.

Vawter, Dorothy E., Warren Kearney, Karen G. Gervais, Arthur L. Caplan, Daniel Garry, and Carol Tauer. *The Use of Human Fetal Tissue: Scientific, Ethical, and Policy Concerns.* Minneapolis: Center for Biomedical Ethics, University of Minnesota, January 1990.

Vawter, Dorothy E., Karen G. Gervais, Warren Kearney, and Arthur L. Caplan. "Fetal Tissue Transplantation and the Problem of Elective Abortion," in *Organ Replacement Therapy: Ethics, Justice, and Commerce,* edited by W. Land and J. B. Dossetor, 492–498. Berlin: Springer-Verlag, 1991.

Weil, William B., and Martin Benjamin, editors. *Ethical Issues at the Onset of Life.* Boston: Blackwell Scientific Publications, 1987.

Winner, Langdon. *The Whale and the Reactor: A Search for Limits in an Age of High Technology.* Chicago: University of Chicago Press, 1986.

JOURNAL AND NEWSPAPER ARTICLES

Adams, B. "Restoring Hope: Lifting the Ban on Fetal Tissue-Transplantation Research." *Academic Medicine* 67, no. 4 (1992), 246–247.

Andrews, Lori B. "My Body, My Property." *Hastings Center Report* 16, no. 5 (October 1986), 28–38.

Annas, George J. "Pregnant Women as Fetal Containers." *Hastings Center Report* 16, no. 6 (December 1986).

Annas, George J., and Sherman Elias. "The Politics of Transplantation of Human Fetal Tissue." *New England Journal of Medicine* 320, no. 16 (20 April 1989), 1079–1082.

Baltimore, David. "Limiting Science: A Biologist's Perspective." *Daedalus* 107, no. 2 (Spring 1978), 37–45.

Blakeslee, Sandra. "Fetal Cell Transplants Show Early Promise in Parkinson Patients." *New York Times,* 12 November 1991, B6.

Boffey, Philip M. "Using Fetal Tissue as a Cure Debated." *New York Times,* 15 September 1988, A31.

Bok, Sissela. "Freedom and Risk." *Daedalus* 107, no. 2 (Spring 1978), 115–127.

Brahams, Diana. "Fetal Spare Parts." *Lancet* 1, no. 8582 (20 February 1988), 424.

Bregman, Jenn S. "Conceiving to Abort and Donate Fetal Tissue: New Ethical Strains in the Transplantation Field: A Survey of Existing Law and a Proposal for Change." *UCLA Law Review* 36, no. 6 (1989), 1167–1205.

Campbell, Courtney S. "Body, Self, and the Property Paradigm." *Hastings Center Report* 22, no. 5 (September–October 1992), 34–42.

Clymer, Adam. "House Vote Lets Stand Ban on Fetal Tissue Research." *New York Times,* 25 June 1992, A19.

Culliton, Barbara J. "Science's Restive Public." *Daedalus* 107, no. 2 (Spring 1978), 147–156.

Field, Nancy E. "Evolving Conceptualization of Property: A Proposal to Decommercialize the Value of Fetal Tissue." *Yale Law Journal* 99, no. 1 (1989), 169–186.

Fine, Alan. "The Ethics of Fetal Tissue Transplants." *Hastings Center Report* 18, no. 3 (June/July 1988), 5–8.

Fletcher, John C., and Mark I. Evans. "Maternal Bonding in Early Fetal Ultrasound Examinations." *New England Journal of Medicine* 308, no. 7 (17 February 1983), 392–393.

Gaylin, Willard, and Marc Lappe. "Fetal Politics." *Atlantic Monthly* (May 1975), 66–71.

Gold, Rachel B., and Dorothy Lehrman. "Fetal Research Under Fire: The Influence of Abortion Politics." *Family Planning Perspectives* 21 (January/February 1989), 6–11.

Goldering, John M. "The Brain-Life Theory: Towards a Consistent Biological Definition of Humanness." *Journal of Medical Ethics* 11, no. 4 (December 1985), 198–204.

Goodlin, R. C. "History of Fetal Monitoring." *American Journal of Obstetrics and Gynecology* 133, no. 3 (February 1979), 323–352.

Greely, Henry T., Thomas Hamm, Rodney Johnson, Carole R. Price, Randy Weingarten, and Thomas Raffin. "Special Report: The Ethical Use of Human Fetal Tissue in Medicine." *New England Journal of Medicine* 320, no. 16 (20 April 1989), 1093–1096.

Hahn, Robert A. "Divisions of Labor: Obstetrician, Women and Society in Williams Obstetrics, 1903–1985." *Medical Anthropology Quarterly* 1, no. 3 (September 1987), 230–282.

Hansen, John T., and John R. Sladek. "Fetal Research." *Science* 246 (1989), 775–779.

Hilts, Philip J. "Anguish Over Medical First: Tissue from Fetus to Fetus." *New York Times,* 16 April 1991, A1, B8.

Hilts, Philip J. "Fetus-to-Fetus Transplant Is Said to Block a Deadly Defect." *New York Times,* 21 November 1991, A14.

Hilts, Philip J. "Congress Urged to Lift Ban on Fetal-Tissue Research." *New York Times,* 27 May 1992, A7.

Holloway, Marguerite. "Fetal Law: Experimental Surgery May Feed Ethical Debates." *Scientific American* (September 1990), 46–47.

Holton, Gerald. "Epilogue to the Issue, 'Limits to Scientific Inquiry'." *Daedalus* 107, no. 2 (Spring 1978), 227–234.

Irwin, Susan, and Brigette Jordan. "Knowledge, Practice, and Power: Court-Ordered Cesarean Sections." *Medical Anthropology Quarterly* 1, no. 3 (September 1987), 319–334.

Johnsen, Dawn E. "The Creation of Fetal Rights: Conflicts with Woman's Constitutional Rights of Liberty, Privacy, and Equal Protection." *Yale Law Journal* 95, no. 3 (January 1986).

Jonas, Hans. "Philosophical Reflections on Experimenting with Human Subjects." *Daedalus* 98 (1969), 219.

Kearney, Warren, Dorothy E. Vawter, and Karen G. Gervais. "Fetal Tissue Research and the Misread Compromise." *Hastings Center Report* 21, no. 5 (September/October 1991), 7–12.

King, Patricia A. "The Juridical Status of the Fetus: A Proposal for Legal Protection of the Unborn." *Michigan Law Review* 77, no. 7 (August 1979), 1976.

King, Patricia A., and Judith Areen. "Legal Regulation of Fetal Tissue Transplantation." *Clinical Research* 36 (April 1988), 205–208.

Kolata, Gina. "More U.S. Curbs Urged in the Use of Fetal Tissue." *New York Times,* 19 November 1989, A1, A38.

Kolata, Gina. "Genetic Defects Detected in Embryos Just Days Old." *New York Times,* 24 September 1992.

Kolata, Gina. "Fetal Ovary Transplant Is Envisioned." *New York Times,* 6 January 1994.

Lenow, Jeffrey L. "The Fetus as a Patient: Emerging Rights as a Person." *American Journal of Law & Medicine* 9, no. 1 (1983), 1–29.

Mahowald, Mary B. "Placing Wedges Along a Slippery Slope: Use of Fetal Neural Tissue for Transplantation." *Clinical Research* 36, no. 3 (1988), 220–222.

McCormick, Richard A. "Experimentation in Children: Sharing in Sociality." *Hastings Center Report* (December 1976), 41–46.

Moussa, Mario, and Thomas A. Shannon. "The Search for the New

Pineal Gland: Brain Life and Personhood." *Hastings Center Report* 22, no. 2 (May–June 1992), 30–37.

Nelkin, Dorothy. "Threats and Promises: Negotiating the Control of Research." *Daedalus* 107, no. 2 (Spring 1978), 191–209.

Nelkin, Dorothy. "The Politics of Personhood." *Health and Society* 61, no. 1 (1983), 101–112.

Noland, Kathleen. "Genug ist Genug: A Fetus Is Not a Kidney." *Hastings Center Report* 18, no. 6 (December 1988), 13–19.

Pollitt, Katha. " 'Fetal Rights': A New Assault on Feminism." *Nation* (26 March 1990), 409–418.

Ramsey, Paul. "The Enforcement of Morals: Nontherapeutic Research on Children." *Hastings Center Report* (August 1976), 21–30.

Scraf, Maggie. "The Fetus as Guinea Pig." *New York Times Magazine,* 19 October 1975, 13.

Sorelle, Ruth. "A Moral Balance: Couple Weighs Abortion Stand Against Own Baby's Vita Need for Fetal Tissue." *Houston Chronicle,* 22 April 1991, 1A, 6A.

Strong, C. "Fetal Tissue-Transplantation: Can It Be Morally Insulated from Abortion." *Journal of Medical Ethics* 17, no. 2 (1991), 70–76.

Toner, Robin. "Clinton Orders Reversal of Abortion Restrictions Left by Reagan and Bush." *New York Times,* 23 January 1993, A1, A7.

Waxman, Henry A. "Research That Could Save Lives." *Washington Post,* 21 May 1991, A-21.

GOVERNMENT DOCUMENTS

Advisory Group to the Department of Health and Social Security, Scottish Home and Health Department and Welsh Office. *The Use of Fetuses and Fetal Material for Research.* London: H.M. Stationery Office, 1972.

Andrews, Lori B. "State Regulation of Human Fetal Tissue Transplantation," in *Report of the Human Fetal Transplantation Research Panel,* edited by Consultants to the Advisory Committee to the Director, vol. II, D1–D20. Washington, DC: National Institutes of Health, 1988.

Bok, Sissela. "Fetal Research and the Value of Life," in *Appendix: Research on the Fetus,* 3–9. Washington, DC: National Commission for the Protection of Human Subjects of Biomedical and Behavioral Research, 1976.

Bush, Vannevar. *Science: The Endless Frontier.* Washington, DC: National Science Foundation, 1960.

U.S. Congress. "Research Freedom Act of 1990," Vol. HR 5456, 18 December 1990.

U.S. Congress, Committee on Energy and Commerce, Subcommittee on Health and the Environment. House of Representatives, 101 Congress, 2nd Session. "Fetal Tissue Transplantation Research," Vol. 101–135. Washington, DC: U.S. Government Printing Office, 2 April 1990.

U.S. Congress, Senate, Committee on Labor and Human Resources. *Finding Medical Cures: The Promise of Fetal Tissue Transplantation Research.* Washington, DC: U.S. Government Printing Office, 1991.

Index